MW01055517

Child Medication Fact Book
for Psychiatric Practice

SECOND EDITION

Joshua Feder, MD

Associate Professor, Infant and Early Childhood Development Program, Fielding Graduate University

Elizabeth Tien, MD

Psychiatrist, Los Angeles County Department of Mental Health

Talia Puzantian, PharmD, BCPP

Professor, Keck Graduate Institute School of Pharmacy, Claremont, CA

Published by Carlat Publishing, LLC
PO Box 626, Newburyport, MA 01950

CARLAT PUBLISHING

Child Medication Fact Book
For Psychiatric Practice, Second Edition

Published by Carlat Publishing, LLC
PO Box 626, Newburyport, MA 01950

Publisher and Editor-in-Chief: Daniel J. Carlat, MD

Deputy Editor: Talia Puzantian, PharmD, BCPP
Executive Editor: Janice Jutras
Senior Editor: Ilana Fogelson
Associate Editor: Harmony Zambrano

Cover illustration by Regina Troyer
Design and layout by Carter Publishing Studio

This CME/CE activity is intended for psychiatrists, developmental and behavioral pediatricians, psychiatric nurses, psychologists, and other health care professionals including primary care providers, with an interest in mental health. The Carlat CME Institute is accredited by the Accreditation Council for Continuing Medical Education to provide continuing medical education for physicians. Carlat CME Institute is approved by the American Psychological Association to sponsor continuing education for psychologists. Carlat CME Institute maintains responsibility for this program and its content. Carlat CME Institute designates this enduring material educational activity for a maximum of eight (8) AMA PRA Category 1 Credits™ or 10 CE for psychologists. Physicians or psychologists should claim credit commensurate only with the extent of their participation in the activity. The American Board of Psychiatry and Neurology has reviewed the *Child Medication Fact Book for Psychiatric Practice* and has approved this program as part of a comprehensive Self-Assessment and CME Program, which is mandated by ABMS as a necessary component of maintenance of certification. CME quizzes must be taken online at www.thecarlatreport.com.

To order, visit www.thecarlatreport.com
or call (866) 348-9279

2 3 4 5 6 7 8 9 10

ISBN #:
Print 979-8-9873354-1-3
Ebook 979-8-9873354-0-6

PRINTED IN THE UNITED STATES OF AMERICA

Table of Contents

Note: Some medications, eg guanfacine, are covered in more than one chapter; however, the fact sheets are listed only in one of those chapters.

Appendices 145

List of Tables

List of Treatment Algorithms

Introduction

HOW TO USE THIS BOOK

We present medication information in four ways:

- *Chapter introductions:* These are guides to general therapeutic categories of child psychopharmacology. There is natural overlap between these areas; however, we hope that our groupings are convenient for quick reference in everyday office practice.
- *Treatment algorithms:* For some specific clinical situations, we created maps to guide you in decision making with an aim to balance efficacy with safety.
- *Quick-scan medication tables:* These are located after the chapter introduction for each therapeutic category and list the very basics: generic and brand names, FDA-approved indications, available strengths, starting doses, and target doses. These tables contain most of the commonly prescribed psychiatric medications in pediatric practice.
- *Medication fact sheets:* In-depth prescribing information for select medications (not all psychiatric medications are covered). There are 76 medication fact sheets in this book. We have included most of the commonly prescribed and newer medications for which there are data and experience in children.

CHANGES AND ADDITIONS TO THE SECOND EDITION

We've updated the medication fact sheets with newer strengths, formulations, generics, and clinical data where available. We have six new fact sheets, five new tables, and two new appendices. We've also added 14 treatment algorithms to this edition where we thought they made sense. Finally, in this edition we made the shift from *treatment* of (person first) autism spectrum *disorder* to *supporting* better function with neurodiverse/*autistic* kids and teens.

CATEGORIES OF MEDICATIONS

We did our best to categorize medications rationally. However, in some cases a medication can fall into more than one therapeutic category. In such cases, we placed the medication's fact sheet in the category for which it is most often used. If you're having trouble finding a medication in a particular section, look in the index to find its page number.

MORE ON THE MEDICATION FACT SHEETS

The goal of these fact sheets is to provide need-to-know information that can be easily and quickly absorbed during a busy day of seeing patients. An important goal, therefore, is that all the information should fit on a single page. Please refer to the *PDR (Physicians' Desk Reference)* when you need more in-depth information.

For the most part, each fact sheet contains the following information:

- Bottom line. We begin with a super-condensed summary, including our overall assessment of the drug's value in clinical practice. If you're in a rush, you can get the very basics from this alone.
- Both the brand and generic names.
- Generic availability, denoted with a [G] or (G).
- FDA-approved indications in kids and in adults.
- Off-label uses. We list the more common off-label uses, based on both the medical literature and our own clinical experience. Just because we list a potential use does not imply that we endorse a medication as being particularly effective in that capacity. We are simply alerting you to the fact that there is some evidence for efficacy or at least reports of use.
- Dosage forms, along with available strengths.
- Dosage guidance. We provide recommendations on how to dose medications; these are derived from a variety of sources, including package inserts, clinical trials, and common clinical practice. In other words, don't be surprised when our dosing instructions are at odds with what you find in the *PDR* or other sources such as RxList.
- Lab monitoring recommendations. We include the usual routine monitoring measures for each medication. Of course, you may need to think beyond the "routine" if the clinical picture warrants it.
- Cost information. Pricing information for a one-month supply of a common dosing regimen was obtained from the website GoodRx (www.goodrx.com), accessed in August 2022. These are the prices patients would have to pay if they had no insurance. Because of wide variations in price depending on the pharmacy, in this edition of the book we list price categories rather than the price in dollars. The categories are:
  - $: Inexpensive: <$50/month
  - $$: Moderate: $50–$100/month
  - $$$: Expensive: $100–$200/month
  - $$$$: Very expensive: $200–$500/month
  - $$$$$: Extremely expensive: >$500/month

  Many patients have insurance and are not going to pay retail, but rather a co-pay, which is usually less expensive. However, off-label uses of medications in child psychiatry are often not covered by insurance. Also, even when medications are covered, their co-pays can be high, particularly for high-deductible insurance plans. With no clear source for accurately predicting a co-pay, you can use the retail price as a clue. Meds that are very inexpensive may require no co-pay, while the most expensive drugs will either require a very expensive co-pay or, more likely, will not be covered at all without an onerous pre-authorization process. We also recommend that families or pharmacies check online for coupon programs such as GoodRx or new companies such as Mark Cuban's CostPlus Drug Company (https://costplusdrugs.com/medications/categories/mental-health/), which frequently offer the same medications at costs far below even the co-pay.

- Side effect information. We break down side effects into "most common" vs "rare but serious" side effects. We generally define "most common" side effects as those that occurred in at least 5% of patients in clinical trials and that occurred at least twice as often compared to the placebo group. Such information is usually found in tables in the drugs' package inserts. We also used post-marketing clinical experience as a guide in determining which side effects were common enough to make the list.
- Mechanism of action. While the mechanism of action is not well established for most psychiatric drugs, we thought it would be important to report the mechanisms most commonly cited.
- Pharmacokinetics, with a focus on drug metabolism and/or half-life.
- Drug interactions.
- Evidence and clinical pearls. These typically comment on the evidence base for use in children and the advantages or disadvantages of a medication in comparison to others in its therapeutic category, tips for dosing or avoiding side effects, types of patients who seem to benefit the most, reports about off-label use, and so forth.
- Fun facts—people tell us that this might be the best part of the book.

APPENDICES

Please note that in these appendices we've included a number of medications that are not generally used in children—we list them anyway for completeness. In the appendices you'll find the following:
- Rating scales. Here we've listed a number of scales that you can use for assessment and tracking, covering autism screening, ADHD, anxiety, and mood problems.
- Abnormal Involuntary Movement Scale (AIMS). While we wish to avoid unneeded use of antipsychotic medications and other drugs that might cause tardive dyskinesia, the AIMS helps us to monitor for such side effects.
- Blood pressure parameters for children. A guide for clinicians, in particular for children on stimulant medications.
- Growth, body mass index, and head circumference charts. These are helpful as we track the growth and development of our patients and monitor for side effects.
- Lab monitoring for psychiatric medications. We've included a short quick-reference table listing the medications that require laboratory monitoring, along with the labs you should consider ordering.
- Informed consent guidelines. This topic can be particularly complicated in child and adolescent psychiatry, so here we've offered guidelines for clinicians to navigate this process.
- Mental health apps. Apps are often really helpful for you or for your patients, if you can tolerate the data privacy concerns. We've listed a few of our favorites.
- Drug interactions in psychiatry. While we've provided some information on drug interactions in the fact sheets, this appendix features a more extensive discussion of the topic, as well as a table of interactions for commonly prescribed drugs.
- Pregnancy and lactation risk information. The risks and benefits of using psychiatric medications in pregnancy and breastfeeding are not as simple or clear as the previously used "ABCDX" categories might suggest. The newer Pregnancy and Lactation Labeling Rule (PLLR) has been implemented by the FDA, resulting in a more detailed narrative describing available risk data instead of the letter category designation. Rather than putting this information in the fact sheets, we've placed a separate section in the appendices devoted to the topic.
- Schedules of controlled substances. Just in case you can't remember which drugs are in which DEA schedule or what each schedule means, we have you covered with a handy table.
- Pharmacogenetic testing recommendations. Although we do not feel that pharmacogenetic testing has reached a stage of routine clinical utility, we've added a brief section providing some basic information.

FINANCIAL DISCLOSURES

Drs. Feder, Tien, and Puzantian have disclosed that they have no relevant relationships or financial interests in any commercial company pertaining to the information provided in this book.

DISCLAIMER

The medication information in this book was formulated with a reasonable standard of care and in conformity with professional standards in the field of child and adolescent psychiatry where available. Medication prescribing decisions are complex, and you should use these fact sheets, tables, and algorithms as only one of many possible sources of medication information. This information is not a substitute for informed medical care. This book is intended for use by licensed professionals only.

If you have any comments or corrections, please let us know by writing to us at info@thecarlatreport.com or Carlat Publishing, PO Box 626, Newburyport, MA 01950.

General Tips on Child and Adolescent Psychopharmacology

Over the course of a career, most of us realize that pediatric psychopharmacology is more art than science, and that much of the knowledge we've acquired over the years has come from our work with patients after completing residency and fellowship. Here are some hard-won tips and pearls that you might find useful in your practice.

ASSESSMENT, DIAGNOSIS, AND CASE CONCEPTUALIZATION

- **Target symptoms are king.** Most patients come to us with mixed symptoms from several diagnostic categories. And many symptoms, such as anxiety, show up in ADHD, depression, autistic kids, and others. So while formal diagnosis is helpful for insurance and school advocacy, for treatment it is usually more practical to list and prioritize target symptoms. During the workup and ongoing follow-up, it is very helpful to have a running list of all the presenting and ongoing target symptoms, circling the ones that are the current focus. For instance, in one patient you might be targeting substance use, mood instability, and impulsivity, circling all three, while leaving issues of poor grades, tics, and peer relationships on the list but uncircled—intending to focus on them a bit down the line. Another patient with the same set of symptoms might have different issues to target.

- **Meds are the tail, not the dog.** Medications can be very helpful at times, even life-saving, but they cannot make up for an inadequate overall plan or placement. If a child is laboring under challenging or outright abusive situations at home or school, pills do not fix that. For instance, an autistic teen was brought in for a medication evaluation for irritability and "acting out." On evaluation, his treatment plan included "training for pre-vocational skills"—and his acting out turned out to be in part a rebellion from years of being subjected to tasks such as sorting silverware. The answer in this case was to rethink the goals that had been imposed on the patient as part of the treatment plan, and not to provide chemical restraint.

- **Informed consent is your friend.** Use informed consent—diagnosis, target symptoms, discussion of options, etc—to guide a rational and ongoing conversation with families. See the appendices for additional tips on this process.

- **Good care demands time.** You know this, and you are probably fighting for time—time to see the patient; talk to family, therapists, and teachers; review records; call labs; and whatever else you need to do to care for your patient. When we are taken to task about care, we are asked such things as: "Did you contact the school?" "Did you call the lab?" We need time to do these things, and we deserve to be paid for that time too. Advocate for more time for all the elements of patient care.

- **Keep development in mind.** One of the joys of our field is that we have the opportunity to see the range of changes that occur developmentally and to explain to parents, teachers, and colleagues that these are not "symptoms." For example, an active toddler does not necessarily have ADHD. A school-aged child with a vivid fantasy life is usually not psychotic.

- **Always consider the possibility of abuse.** It is estimated that 1/4 to 1/3 of girls and 1/6 of boys are sexually abused before age 18; always assess for sexual and physical abuse as well as neglect. Ask about discipline and supervision as a part of your formal assessment. Parents often want help in managing their frustration (and perhaps their own difficulties with mood, substances, etc), and this is an opportunity to be of great assistance.

- **Drug and substance use are common.** We should always ask teens (and even tweens) about substance use. This includes the usual things like tobacco, alcohol, marijuana, and other drugs; prescribed medications such as stimulants and opiates; over-the-counter medications such as dextromethorphan, antihistamines, and pseudoephedrine; readily available inhalants such as glue, gasoline, and many others; non-prescribed opiates; CBD; and newer drugs of abuse. In addition, consider substances not yet or newly criminalized such as kratom, spice, and others. As of this writing, fentanyl is killing more and more kids, laced into marijuana, heroin, and many kinds of faked pills including opiates such as OxyContin, stimulants such as Adderall, and benzodiazepines such as Xanax.

- **We may save more lives with a safety check than anything else we do.** Talk with parents about locking up alcohol, medications (including over-the-counter meds), and hazardous household products. We often add an admonition to lock up or remove guns, ropes, cords, and sharp knives from homes as part of a safety check. Ask about sunscreen, hydration, seat belts, and driving habits of the patient and the family. Natural disasters are becoming more common. Asking about the family's fire, earthquake, and tsunami plans makes sense for proactive health care providers.

MEDICATION MANAGEMENT AND MONITORING TARGET SYMPTOMS

- **Change one thing at a time.** Try to make only one medication change at a time. Starting two medications at once, for example, can make it hard to tell which one is easing symptoms and which one is causing side effects. There will be exceptions, particularly in more urgent situations; however, it is best to try to be parsimonious and patient.

- **Start low and go slow.** While making small changes may take patience and reassurance, rapid or large changes in medications often lead to untoward side effects and aborted medication trials. It is helpful to tell families, especially if they are hesitant about medication, that we want to use the lowest effective dose; therefore, the best first result is to see no change in symptoms and no side effects because we've used so little medication. From here, we bring up the dose gradually so we can see the results.

- **Treat with the end in mind. Medication is a means to an end, not an end in itself. How long makes sense? For most medications, we do not have data to show that long-term use is helpful.** There is little point in keeping a medication at a robust dose if it is not having a clear positive impact. We often see people who have stayed on medications more out of habit than anything else. Get rid of unneeded medications, but do it gradually. The medication may in fact be helping, or perhaps a combination is important (eg, in classic bipolar disorder). Even if the medication is not helping, your patient might suffer severe discontinuation symptoms if you stop it too quickly, which will further confuse the issue.

- **Beware regression to the mean.** We often see people when things are difficult; however, many symptoms will wax and wane as part of their natural course. If we start a medication when a particular symptom is at its worst, we may ascribe the subsequent improvement to our intervention when the symptom would have gotten better anyway. The reverse is also true: When a symptom worsens, we may automatically attribute it to a life event or to a medication change.

- **Placebo effects are common.** Hope and faith are good things and might bring about positive results from an otherwise ineffective medication. If a positive response diminishes after about six weeks, it may have been mostly a placebo effect.

- **Beware polypharmacy.** Sometimes we prescribe combinations of medications more as a way to deal with our own anxieties about a difficult case than as a response to research-driven, evidence-based guidelines. Try to clarify the rationale for the medication regimen and document your thinking.

- **Some patients may need microdosing.** Some patients respond best to tiny doses of a medication (eg, as little as a milligram of an SSRI). It's worth trying in patients who are unable to tolerate higher doses. This may or may not track with pharmacogenetic findings.

- **Other patients may need megadosing.** Some patients seem to require higher-than-usual doses of a medication. If you embark on a high-dose regimen, look for supporting literature (research, case studies), take great care and time in the process, and keep clear documentation. This too may or may not track with pharmacogenetic findings.

- **Perform physiological follow-up.** Be scrupulous about monitoring for potential side effects. Depending on the drug, this may include tracking growth, vital signs, indicated labs, neurological checks such as the Abnormal Involuntary Movement Scale (AIMS) for patients on antipsychotics, ECGs, etc. Don't assume that the patient's primary care provider will keep up with these tests. Our patients are less likely to have good primary and preventative care overall, much less good follow-up for the effects of our prescriptions. Check the appendices for some helpful resources.

- **Don't skimp on visits.** Patients and their families often give compelling reasons for avoiding follow-up visits. Push back a little. Soccer practice is important, but medical care is more important. If you determine that it is legal and clinically appropriate, see college kids as you would any patient that age, or arrange for them to receive care near their campus.

- **Weigh in-person vs telehealth visits.** Is your patient alone and able to talk freely from home? Do you need to do a more thorough neurological screen than what you can guide the patient to do over internet video? What's the risk of coming in vs the convenience of staying home? Is an outdoor appointment an option? Welcome to the age of the pandemic.

- **Make use of rating scales.** Accurate assessment and outcomes matter. We need to find ways to support our assessment process and track symptoms using validated scales. Rating scales cannot replace good clinical follow-up, but they can be helpful for supporting our diagnostic thinking, uncovering problems, or getting us to think about and document why we might not agree with the scale. In this edition we've listed some of our favorites in Appendix A, picked for their validity, ease of use, and low cost.

- **Stay patient, thoughtful, and steady.** Families may be tempted to quit medication trials too soon, but we need to remind them that medications take time to work, and that side effects often fade after a few days or can be addressed with medication adjustments or other strategies.

QUICK REVIEW OF DEVELOPMENTAL ASSESSMENT AND PSYCHOPHARMACOLOGY

Infants and Young Children

- **Assess young children through their interactions.** Young children often demonstrate their functional abilities and challenges best through their interactions with parents and caregivers. Observe them during these interactions, not when they are isolated in your office. It is also helpful to observe children in other settings (by video or video recording if needed) such as at the home, preschool, park, etc. Early childhood mental health is a field of its own, and if you aren't trained or experienced in this field, you deserve support from colleagues.

- **Pharmacodynamic and pharmacokinetic processes differ in infants.** Drug metabolism and brain effects change from neonate to infant to child to adolescent. Infants and younger children have reduced absorption, plasma protein binding, hepatic metabolism, and both renal and gastrointestinal (pancreatic-mediated) excretion. Higher brain-to-body weight and immaturity of brain development can also affect the efficacy of psychotropic medications. CYP metabolism is at about 50%–70% of adult levels in young children. For any medication, dosing may require higher or lower mg/kg than for adults. Common examples include stimulants' relative lack of efficacy and more frequent side effects, and the significantly higher toxicity of valproic acid in very young children. For any use of psychotropic medications in young children, it is important to double-check dosing guidelines specific to this population.

School-Aged Children

- **School-aged kids may need to stay out of the room while you have frank discussions with caregivers.** Parents need to tell you what their children are doing, yet this can be a humiliating experience when the child is present. Try to schedule times to talk with parents by themselves. This may require arranging a safe care setting for the child, but it is well worth the effort.
- **School-aged kids often have trouble talking.** School-aged kids may not talk about their issues. Their symptoms may become apparent during games, drawing, or other activities. Observation may reveal symptoms such as inattentiveness, trouble reading, expecting defeat, etc. You might try to talk with children about symptoms, but don't press them or shame them for not not "opening up." They might not be able to talk about feelings. Collateral data from caregivers, teachers, and others are essential. Sources that agree can confirm your diagnostic thinking. Sources that differ (eg, anxious in one setting but not another) beg investigation.
- **Be concrete with school-aged children.** Children may not report specific difficulties unless you ask them explicitly and use words they understand. They may be very suggestible as well, so yes-or-no questions may require follow-up. "How tired are you? A little? A lot? Is it making things different for you?"
- **Consider the liver.** CYP metabolism, while low in early childhood, may be higher than adult levels in middle childhood and may result in a need for higher doses than expected. As always, start low and go slow. Hepatic efficiency typically falls to adult levels with puberty, so some medication doses may need to be reduced, both to alleviate side effects and to use the lowest effective dose.
- **Take SSRI side effects into account.** There may be relatively high rates of behavioral activation with SSRIs, with many proposed mechanisms including serotonergic differences in children. Take this into account initially and in follow-up.
- **Let hormones do their jobs.** We often attribute some of the difficulties of tweens and teens to pubertal changes in hormones and the accompanying social and psychological shifts. It's true. Don't try to medicate normal developmental changes—instead, encourage caregivers to manage these changes via empathic developmental and behavioral strategies.

Teens

- **Teens often do worse when we leave them in the waiting room.** Managing appointments can become a round robin of seeing the parent and child together, the child alone, the parent alone, etc. Teens often do not do well if we leave them in the waiting room while we talk to caregivers. They expect and require more confidentiality and ownership of the doctor-patient relationship. Sitting in the waiting room, they are left stewing, possibly making assumptions about what is being discussed. In such cases, try to get your updates from parents via phone calls or emails, rather than checking in during the teen's appointment.
- **Teens are not quite young adults.** Teens often have an entirely different manner of processing information and assessing risk than adults. Do not let their adult appearance lead you to presume that they can competently weigh the risks and benefits of treatments and daily decisions. As a rule, teens will minimize risks. They also tend to prefer being out in the world rather than showing up for appointments. Meanwhile, those who actually *want* to come to see us may well be suffering more severely than they let on.
- **Adult-ish dosing is generally OK.** Physiologically speaking, most teens can use doses that we typically use in adults.
- **Teens often miss medication.** Teens often miss doses of their medication and may be concurrently using other substances. It is important to acknowledge and normalize these behaviors to reduce shame. Ask teens directly whether they have missed medications and whether they have tried any other substances lately. Sometimes medications with longer half-lives (eg, fluoxetine) make sense in order to minimize the effects of missed doses.
- **Use supervision and avoid diversion.** More than any other intervention, good supervision is important in the overall plan for teens. While many become able to manage their own medications (and should be taught medication management before going off to college), most need parental guidance and often parental doling out of daily or weekly doses. Keeping parents involved also reduces drug diversion, as long as parents themselves are not using the medications. Close parental monitoring of medication is especially important for teens who are overdose risks.

CLOSING THOUGHT: DON'T DO THIS ALONE

Prescribing for children is challenging. You can't think of everything, and it is important to have access to trusted colleagues and to be part of an ongoing process of case discussion and mutual support. Our field is constantly changing, and the best way to stay on top of the changes is to be engaged in a continual conversation about what we do and how we do it.

ADHD Medications

Generally, in treating kids with ADHD, you should start with psychostimulants, since they are the most effective options. Second-line agents include alpha-agonists, followed by atomoxetine, viloxazine, and bupropion.

STIMULANT RECOMMENDATIONS

When choosing a stimulant, the first decision is between an amphetamine or methylphenidate preparation. More recent data have suggested that, based on safety and efficacy, methylphenidates are a better choice in kids and adolescents whereas amphetamine-class agents are better in adults. Yet, even in adults, we generally recommend going with a methylphenidate preparation first based on lower side effect and misuse potential. The second decision is choosing between a long-acting or short-acting stimulant.

For kids who don't like swallowing pills, there are various options. Some long-acting stimulants can be opened and sprinkled on food. There are also short- and long-acting liquid, chewable, and disintegrating brand-name options—though they are expensive and often require pre-authorization. Finally, another option for the pill-phobics is the Daytrana or Xelstrym patch.

When initiating a trial of stimulant medication, titrating the dose on a weekly basis optimizes the response efficiently, with the added benefit of limiting the use of additional medications with their associated side effects. While valproate and risperidone have been demonstrated to be effective for aggression with ADHD, you will rarely need them if you prioritize stimulant titration.

The Case for Long-Acting Stimulants

- More practical: It's easier to take a single dose that lasts through the duration of a school day.
- Addresses acute tachyphylaxis: Response to stimulants diminishes rapidly, but most newer long-acting stimulants release an increasing amount of drug over the dose's six- to 12-hour course, which most people need for the medication to be effective. This avoids the need for multiple short-acting dosage bursts to maintain continued response.
- Decreased stimulant rebound: People sensitive to rebound irritability or worsening of ADHD symptoms often report a more attenuated rebound with long-acting stimulants.

The Case for Short-Acting Stimulants

- For situations where a child only requires a few hours of effect, such as a half day of school, an afternoon of completing homework, or a weekend activity.
- Minimizes appetite suppression during meals.
- May be less likely to interfere with sleep.

DOSE EQUIVALENTS

Some kids may need to try different stimulants, or stimulant formulations, before settling on the one that works best for them. The dose equivalents are, luckily, fairly easy to remember.

1. **From one amphetamine to another amphetamine**
   - With the exception of Vyvanse, all amphetamines, including Adderall IR and XR, are roughly equivalent in potency. For example, if a child is taking Dexedrine 10 mg TID, you can switch this to Adderall 15 mg BID or Adderall XR 30 mg QD. That said, some people believe that Dexedrine, being 100% dextroamphetamine, might be more potent than Adderall, which is 75% d-amphetamine and 25% l-amphetamine (eg, Dexedrine 30 mg/day may be closer to 40 mg/day of Adderall). In reality, the effect is likely negligible in most people.
   - Vyvanse is composed of both lysine and amphetamine, with amphetamine making up only about 30% of the drug. This means that Vyvanse is much less potent than straight Dexedrine. So when switching from another amphetamine to Vyvanse, you have to at least *double the dose*, and sometimes more.

2. **From one methylphenidate to another methylphenidate**
   - With the exception of Concerta and Focalin, all methylphenidate preparations are roughly equivalent in potency.
   - Concerta, because of its complex delivery system, delivers less methylphenidate than implied by the mg amount you prescribe. The usual conversion percentage used is 83%, meaning that the body sees 83% of Concerta in methylphenidate equivalents. Thus, Concerta 18 mg is equivalent to methylphenidate 15 mg, 36 mg is equivalent to 30 mg, and so on.
   - Focalin is the dextro-isomer of methylphenidate, which is twice as potent as methylphenidate. Thus, use about half the dose when using Focalin.

3. **From a methylphenidate to an amphetamine (or vice versa)**
   - Methylphenidate is roughly half as potent as amphetamine, so Ritalin 10 mg = Dexedrine 5 mg, etc. Consistent with this equivalency, child psychiatrists often dose methylphenidate at 1 mg/kg/immediate-release dose, whereas they dose amphetamine at 0.5 mg/kg. Conversely, if you're switching from Dexedrine to Ritalin, you would need to double the dosage.

4. **From an oral methylphenidate to the methylphenidate patch (Daytrana)**
   - According to a clinical trial of kids switched from various versions of long-acting methylphenidate to the patch, you should dose the patch at about half the dose of the oral medication.

5. **From an oral amphetamine to the dextroamphetamine patch (Xelstrym)**
   - As Xelstrym is a newer formulation, the recommendation is to titrate the patch dose from the usual starting dose rather than approximate an equivalent substitution dose.

HOW TO SWITCH

Once you've determined the dose equivalence, the actual switching is easy. Don't cross-taper; just have your patient take the last dose of stimulant A on day 1 and start stimulant B on day 2. To be prudent, start the new stimulant at a somewhat lower dose than the calculation you arrived at via the equivalent dose guideline. Those equivalencies are based on averages and may not apply to a given individual.

HOW TO STOP

When discontinuing stimulant medications, no taper is required; the medications can just be stopped given their fast action and metabolism. The same is not true for the longer-acting non-stimulant options—especially alpha-agonists, which should be tapered to avoid rebound hypertension. The bigger question is *when* to stop. About a third of young patients seem to do OK letting go of stimulants in their late teens or early 20s. Others stop due to side effects, perhaps trying non-stimulant options.

NON-STIMULANT RECOMMENDATIONS

Although their efficacy cannot compare to stimulants, atomoxetine or viloxazine may be an appropriate first step when you're concerned about diversion or substance misuse. For children with severe tic disorders, guanfacine and clonidine may be indicated with the added benefit of targeting the tics. Alpha-agonists are also helpful for addressing the frequent sleep difficulties found in children with ADHD. Patients with comorbid depression or tobacco use may benefit from bupropion. A handful of clinical trials suggest that modafinil may be an option when stimulant response is limited. Regardless of your choice, don't expect the robust and rapid response frequently seen with stimulants.

Some studies have demonstrated small improvements in ADHD symptoms with higher doses of omega-3, specifically eicosapentaenoic acid (EPA), as a supplement; however, this has not been consistently supported in meta-analyses. Limited evidence also exists for ginkgo biloba and saffron in reducing ADHD symptoms. While these should not replace the use of a stimulant or non-stimulant medication, they may be useful as an adjunct and for families who are not currently interested in medication options.

Lastly, the FDA approved a medical device, the Monarch external trigeminal nerve stimulation (eTNS) system, for children 7–12 years of age based off a single small four-week study. The cost remains significant for an option that lacks solid data. There is also an FDA-approved videogame called EndeavorRx for treatment of ADHD. Wonders never cease.

STIMULANT SIDE EFFECTS AND CLASS WARNINGS

- The most common side effects include appetite suppression and insomnia. With long-term use, due to chronic appetite suppression and acute growth hormone inhibition, some literature has reported an average decrease of half an inch in expected height, while several studies have not found significant differences with longer-term follow-up or "drug holidays." Despite this, drug holidays are still useful on weekends and school breaks for patients who struggle with appropriate weight gain, assuming their behavioral functioning remains manageable without medication. Taking stimulant medication with or after breakfast, providing snacks throughout the day, and scheduling a high-caloric evening snack when appetite has bounced back can help to manage appetite suppression, related irritability, and weight loss. High-caloric and protein milkshakes or smoothies with some combination of Ensure, whole milk, yogurt, milk powder, fruit, peanut butter, and ice cream can be on the menu. Cyproheptadine is sometimes used, but studies are limited. Additionally, stimulants should be avoided in patients with anorexia nervosa given their GI and anorectic side effects.

- Stimulants have been known to unmask underlying tics, and at times they can exacerbate an established Tourette's or tic disorder. To complicate matters further, most children present for ADHD treatment during the age range when tics begin to manifest and worsen. For patients with more severe tics, alpha-agonists are worth considering prior to a stimulant trial.

- In patients with a seizure disorder, stimulants may lower the seizure threshold, although the current data are contradictory.

- In patients with a genetic predisposition to or history of psychosis, stimulants can exacerbate symptoms in a dose-dependent fashion. Amphetamine products have at least double the psychosis risk of methylphenidate products.
- Patients with a comorbid anxiety disorder may experience a worsening of anxiety symptoms; however, anxiety and also boredom may improve.
- Research has debunked prior concerns that stimulants might not work as well and produce more side effects in autistic children and teens.
- Some patients have been known to have increased skin picking, hair pulling, and nail biting behaviors with stimulant medications. Alpha-agonists may be helpful here too.
- A few patients may experience an increase in aggressive behaviors or other adverse psychiatric effects (hallucinations, delusions, mania).
- Stimulants may increase heart rate and blood pressure, particularly in older patients; thus, vitals should be monitored at baseline and with subsequent dose adjustments. Blood pressure parameters vary in children by age, height, and sex (see Appendix C). Patients with cardiovascular symptoms, with a family history of early cardiac death or cardiac arrhythmias, or who are adopted with unknown family histories would benefit from additional consultation from their primary care physician or cardiologist.
- Black box warnings for abuse and dependence: Patients with a history of recent substance use should be followed more closely if stimulants are considered, given the risk of diversion, overuse, and dependence of these medications. Vyvanse is thought to have decreased misuse potential due to being a prodrug that becomes active only after oral ingestion.

ADHD Treatment Algorithm for Children and Adolescents

*Denotes off label

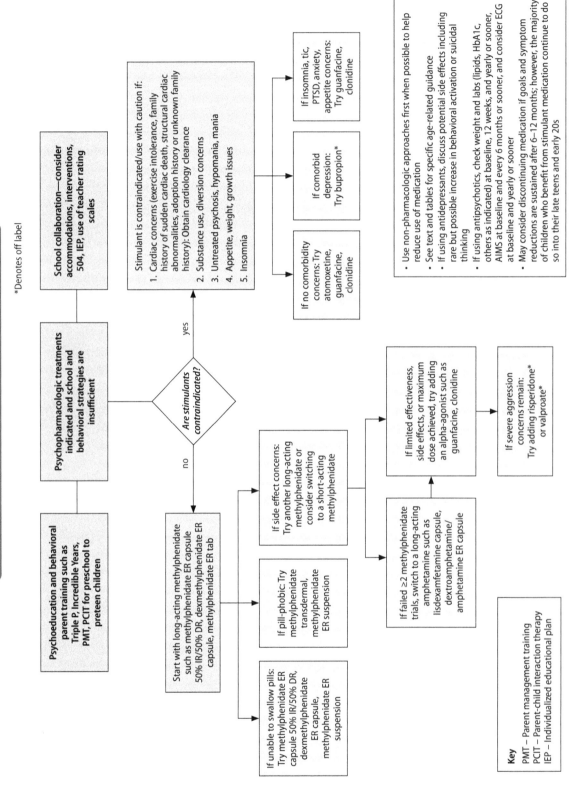

Psychoeducation and behavioral parent training such as Triple P, Incredible Years, PMT, PCIT for preschool to preteen children

Psychopharmacologic treatments indicated and school and behavioral strategies are insufficient

School collaboration—consider accommodations, interventions, 504, IEP, use of teacher rating scales

Are stimulants contraindicated?

no

yes

Start with long-acting methylphenidate such as methylphenidate ER capsule 50% IR/50% DR, dexmethylphenidate ER capsule, methylphenidate ER tab

If unable to swallow pills: Try methylphenidate ER capsule 50% IR/50% DR, dexmethylphenidate ER capsule, methylphenidate ER suspension

If pill-phobic: Try methylphenidate transdermal, methylphenidate ER suspension

If side effect concerns: Try another long-acting methylphenidate or consider switching to a short-acting methylphenidate

If failed ≥2 methylphenidate trials, switch to a long-acting amphetamine such as lisdexamfetamine capsule, dextroamphetamine/amphetamine ER capsule

If limited effectiveness, side effects, or maximum dose achieved, try adding an alpha-agonist such as guanfacine, clonidine

If severe aggression concerns remain: Try adding risperidone* or valproate*

Stimulant is contraindicated/use with caution if:
1. Cardiac concerns (exercise intolerance, family history of sudden cardiac death, structural cardiac abnormalities, adoption history or unknown family history): Obtain cardiology clearance
2. Substance use, diversion concerns
3. Untreated psychosis, hypomania, mania
4. Appetite, weight, growth issues
5. Insomnia

If no comorbidity concerns: Try atomoxetine, guanfacine, clonidine

If comorbid depression: Try bupropion*

If insomnia, tic, PTSD, anxiety, appetite concerns: Try guanfacine, clonidine

- Use non-pharmacologic approaches first when possible to help reduce use of medication
- See text and tables for specific age-related guidance
- If using antidepressants, discuss potential side effects including rare but possible increase in behavioral activation or suicidal thinking
- If using antipsychotics, check weight and labs (lipids, HbA1c, others as indicated) at baseline, 12 weeks, and yearly or sooner, AIMS at baseline and every 6 months or sooner, and consider ECG at baseline and yearly or sooner
- May consider discontinuing medication if goals and symptom reductions are sustained after 6–12 months; however, the majority of children who benefit from stimulant medication continue to do so into their late teens and early 20s

Key
PMT – Parent management training
PCIT – Parent-child interaction therapy
IEP – Individualized educational plan

TABLE 1: ADHD Medications

Brand Name (Generic Name, if different than heading) Year FDA Approved [G] denotes generic availability	Available Strengths (mg except where noted)	Usual Pediatric Dosage Range (starting–max) (mg)	Onset of Action (minutes)	Duration of Action (hours)	Can It Be Split?	Ages Approved for ADHD	Delivery System/Notes (IR = immediate release, CR = controlled release, DR = delayed release, ER = extended release)
Methylphenidates							
Short-acting							
Focalin [G] (Dexmethylphenidate) 2001	2.5, 5, 10	2.5–10 BID	30–45	3–4	Yes (not scored)	6–17	Tablet; D-enantiomer of Ritalin; 2x more potent than methylphenidate
Methylin CT [G] 2003	2.5, 5, 10	2.5 BID–20 TID	30–45	3–4	Yes	6–17, adults	Chewable, grape-flavored tablet
Methylin oral solution [G] 2002	5 mg/5 mL, 10 mg/5 mL	2.5 BID–20 TID	30–45	3–4	N/A (liquid)	6–17, adults	Clear, grape-flavored liquid
Ritalin [G] 1955	5, 10, 20	2.5 BID–20 TID	30–45	3–4	Yes	6–17, adults	IR tablet
Intermediate-acting							
Metadate ER [G] Branded generic of Ritalin SR 1999	20	10 QAM–30 BID (max 60/day)	60–90	6–8	No	6–17, adults	CR tablet (less predictable because of wax matrix)
Methylin ER [G] Branded generic of Ritalin SR 2000	10, 20	20–60 QAM	60–90	4–8	No	6–17, adults	Hydrophilic polymer tablet; possibly more continuous than others in category
Ritalin SR [G] 1982	10, 20	10–60 QAM	60–90	4–8	No	6–17, adults	CR tablet (less predictable because of wax matrix)
Long-acting							
Adhansia XR 2019	25, 35, 45, 55, 70, 85	25–85 QAM	45–60	10–16	Can be sprinkled; do not crush or chew	6–17, adults	Capsule of 20% IR beads & 80% DR beads
Aptensio XR 2015	10, 15, 20, 30, 40, 50, 60	10–60 QAM	45–60	8–12	Can be sprinkled; do not crush or chew	6–17, adults	Capsule of 40% IR beads & 60% DR beads
Azstarys (Serdexmethylphenidate/ dexmethylphenidate) 2021	26.1/5.2, 39.2/7.8, 52.3/10.4	39.2/7.8– 52.3/10.4 QAM	30–60	8–13	Can be sprinkled or added to water	6–17, adults	Combination of prodrug of dexmethylphenidate (70%) and d-MPH (30%); equivalent to 20, 30, 40 mg dexmethylphenidate (Focalin); twice as potent as methylphenidate
Concerta [G] 2000	18, 27, 36, 54	18–72 QAM	45–60	10–12	No	6–17, adults	CR tablet with 22% IR & 78% DR

Brand Name (Generic Name, if different than heading) Year FDA Approved [G] denotes generic availability	Available Strengths (mg except where noted)	Usual Pediatric Dosage Range (starting–max) (mg)	Onset of Action (minutes) / Duration of Action (hours)		Can It Be Split?	Ages Approved for ADHD	Delivery System/Notes (IR = immediate release, CR = controlled release, DR = delayed release, ER = extended release)
Cotempla XR-ODT 2017	8.6, 17.3, 25.9	17.3–51.8 QAM	45–60	8–12	No (ODT)	6–17	Orally disintegrating, ER with 25% IR & 75% ER
Daytrana patch (Methylphenidate transdermal system) 2006	10, 15, 20, 30	10–30 QAM Remove after 9 hours	120	8–12	No	6–17	CR patch; duration can be shortened by decreasing wear time; drug effects may persist for 5 hours after removal
Focalin XR [G] (Dexmethylphenidate XR) 2005	5, 10, 15, 20, 25, 30, 35, 40	5–30 QAM	30	8–12	Can be sprinkled; do not crush or chew	6–17, adults	Capsule of 50% IR beads & 50% DR beads; mimics BID dosing; 2x more potent than methylphenidate
Jornay PM 2018	20, 40, 60, 80, 100	20–100 QPM	8–10 hrs	8–12; after 10-hr delay in onset	Can be sprinkled; do not crush or chew	6–17, adults	ER capsule of DR beads; taken in evening between 6:30–9:30 pm
Metadate CD [G] 2001	10, 20, 30, 40, 50, 60	20–60 QAM	60–90	8–12	Can be sprinkled; do not crush or chew	6–17, adults	Capsule of 30% IR beads & 70% DR beads; mimics BID dosing
Quillichew ER 2015	20, 30, 40	20–60 QAM	45–60	8–12	Yes	6–17, adults	Chewable ER for those who will not swallow pills or take liquid; 30% IR & 70% ER
Quillivant XR 2012	25 mg/5 mL	20–60 QAM	45	8–12	N/A (liquid)	6–17, adults	20% IR & 80% ER in oral solution; shake prior to use
Ritalin LA [G] 2002	10, 20, 30, 40, 60	20–60 QAM	60–90	8–12	Can be sprinkled; do not crush or chew	6–17, adults	Capsule of 50% IR beads & 50% DR beads
Amphetamines							
Short-acting							
Desoxyn [G] (Methamphetamine) 1943	5	5 QAM–10 BID	30–45	3–5	Yes (scored)	6–17	Tablet
Dexedrine [G] (Dextroamphetamine) 1976	5, 10	3–5 yrs: 2.5 QAM–20 BID; 6–16 yrs: 5 QAM–20 BID	30–45	3–5	Yes	3–16	Scored tablet
Evekeo Evekeo ODT (Amphetamine) 2012, 2019	5, 10 ODT: 2.5, 5, 10, 15, 20	3–5 yrs: 2.5 QAM–20 BID; 6–17 yrs: 5 QAM–20 BID	30–45	3–5	Yes (scored) No (ODT)	3–17	Scored tablet or ODT; 1:1 ratio of l- and d-amphetamine

Brand Name (Generic Name, if different than heading) Year FDA Approved [G] denotes generic availability	Available Strengths (mg except where noted)	Usual Pediatric Dosage Range (starting–max) (mg)	Onset of Action (minutes) / Duration of Action (hours)	Can It Be Split?	Ages Approved for ADHD	Delivery System/Notes (IR = immediate release, CR = controlled release, DR = delayed release, ER = extended release)
ProCentra [G] (Dextroamphetamine oral solution) 2008	5 mg/5 mL	5–20 BID	30–45 / 3–5	N/A (liquid)	3–16	Bubblegum-flavored liquid
Zenzedi (Dextroamphetamine) 2013	2.5, 5, 7.5, 10, 15, 20, 30	3–5 yrs: 2.5–20 BID; 6–16 yrs: 5 QAM–20 BID (same as Dexedrine dosing)	30–45 / 3–5	Yes	3–16	Tablet; 5 mg scored, 10 mg double scored, rest unscored
Intermediate-acting						
Adderall [G] (Mixed amphetamine salts) 1960	5, 7.5, 10, 12.5, 15, 20, 30	3–5 yrs: 2.5 QAM–20 BID; 6–17 yrs: 5 QAM–20 BID	45–60 / 6–8	Can be crushed	3–17, adults	Tablet; mixed salt of l- and d-amphetamine
Long-acting						
Adderall XR [G] (Mixed amphetamine salts) 2001	5, 10, 15, 20, 25, 30	6–12 yrs: 5–30 QAM; 13–17 yrs: 10–40 QAM	45–60 / 8–12	Can be sprinkled; do not crush or chew	6–17, adults	Capsule of 50% IR beads & 50% DR beads; mixed salt of l- and d-amphetamine; mimics BID dosing
Adzenys XR-ODT Adzenys ER oral suspension (Amphetamine) 2016, 2017	3.1, 6.3, 9.4, 12.5, 15.7, 18.8 Oral suspension: 1.25 mg/mL	6–12 yrs: 6.3–18.8 QAM; 13–17 yrs: 6.3–12.5 QAM	45–60 / 8–12	No (ODT, liquid)	6–17, adults	ER orally disintegrating tablets; 3.1 mg is equivalent to 5 mg mixed salts product; increasing dose preparations are equivalent to 10 mg, 15 mg, 20 mg, 25 mg, and 30 mg respectively. Solution: 1.25 mg is equivalent to 2 mg Adderall XR.
Dexedrine Spansules [G] (Dextroamphetamine) 1976	5, 10, 15	5 QAM–20 BID	30–60 / 6–8	Can be sprinkled; do not crush or chew	3–16	Capsule of 50% IR & 50% sustained-release beads
Dyanavel XR (Amphetamine) 2015, 2021	5, 10, 15, 20 Oral suspension: 2.5 mg/mL	2.5–20 QAM	45–60 / 8–12	No (oral suspension)	6–17	ER oral suspension allowing once-daily dosing (must shake well); 2.5 mg = 4 mg mixed amphetamine salts
Mydayis (Mixed amphetamine salts) 2017	12.5, 25, 37.5, 50	12.5–25 QAM	45–60 / 10–16	Can be sprinkled; do not crush or chew	13–17, adults	pH-dependent ER capsule formulation; may have effect up to 16 hours
Vyvanse (Lisdexamfetamine) 2007, 2017	10, 20, 30, 40, 50, 60, 70 Chewable: 10, 20, 30, 40, 50, 60	30–70 QAM	60–90 / 8–13	Can be dissolved in water or sprinkled into soft food	6–17, adults	Lisdexamfetamine is prodrug of dextroamphetamine
Xelstrym patch (Dextroamphetamine transdermal system) 2022	4.5, 9, 13.5, 18	4.5 QAM–18 QAM Remove after 9 hours	120 / 8–12	No	6–17, adults	CR patch; duration can be shortened by decreasing wear time; drug effects may persist for 5 hours after removal

Brand Name (Generic Name, if different than heading) Year FDA Approved [G] denotes generic availability	Available Strengths (mg except where noted)	Usual Pediatric Dosage Range (starting–max) (mg)	Onset of Action (minutes)	Duration of Action (hours)	Can It Be Split?	Ages Approved for ADHD	Delivery System/Notes (IR = immediate release, CR = controlled release, DR = delayed release, ER = extended release)
Non-stimulants							
Catapres [G] (Clonidine IR) 1974	0.1, 0.2, 0.3 Patch: 0.1/day, 0.2/day, 0.3/day	0.05 QHS; increase by 0.05 mg/day every 3–7 days and give divided up to QID; max 0.4 QD	N/A	4–6 (tablets); 24 (patch)	Tablets can be crushed	Not FDA approved for ADHD; approved for adults 18+ for hypertension	Avoid abrupt discontinuation; taper slowly over 4–7 days to reduce risk of rebound hypertension
Intuniv [G] (Guanfacine ER) 2009	1, 2, 3, 4	1–4 QD (do not increase faster than 1 mg/wk) (adolescents 7 mg/day max)	N/A	24	No	6–17	ER tablet; do not stop abruptly (rebound hypertension); not a 1:1 conversion from IR; do not give with high-fat meals
Kapvay [G] (Clonidine XR) 2010	0.1, 0.2	0.1 QHS; increase by 0.1 mg/day weekly and give divided BID; max 0.4 QD	N/A	12–16	No	6–17	ER tablet; titrate gradually (orthostatic hypotension); avoid abrupt discontinuation; somnolence
Provigil [G] (Modafinil) 1998	100, 200	100–400 QAM	N/A	18–24	Yes (200 mg tabs are scored)	Not FDA approved for ADHD	Tablet; studies have shown modafinil to be helpful for ADHD, but low incidence of serious rash; minimal data in children
Qelbree (Viloxazine ER) 2021	100, 150, 200	100–400 QAM	N/A	24	Can be sprinkled	6–17, adults	ER capsule; norepinephrine reuptake inhibitor
Strattera [G] (Atomoxetine) 2002	10, 18, 25, 40, 60, 80, 100	Dosage varies[1]	N/A	24	No	6–17, adults	Capsule; norepinephrine reuptake inhibitor
Tenex [G] (Guanfacine IR) 1986	1, 2	1–4 QD (do not increase faster than 1 mg/wk)	N/A	17	Can be crushed	Not FDA approved for kids or ADHD; approved only for adults 18+ for hypertension	Avoid abrupt discontinuation; taper slowly over 4–7 days to reduce risk of rebound hypertension
Wellbutrin [G] (Bupropion) 1985	75, 100	1.4–6 mg/kg/day	N/A	6–9	Yes	Not FDA approved for ADHD	Tablet; bupropion SR and XL versions exist

[1]Strattera dosing: Weight <70 kg, start 0.5 mg/kg, target 1.2 mg/kg, max 1.4 mg/kg; weight >70 kg, 40–100 mg

TABLE 2: Relative Equivalency and Conversion Guide for Stimulants[1]

Methylphenidates	
Alternative Formulation	**Regular Methylphenidate Equivalent**
Adhansia XR 25 mg QAM	5 mg IR TID
Adhansia XR 50 mg QAM	10 mg IR TID
Aptensio XR 10 mg QAM	5 mg IR BID or 10 mg ER QAM
Concerta 18, 27, 36, 54 mg tablets	10–15, 15–20, 20–30, 30–45 mg/day, respectively; use 72 mg Concerta for 45–60 mg/day
Cotempla XR-ODT 8.6, 17.3, 25.9 mg tablets	ER 10, 20, 30 mg, respectively
Daytrana patch 10 mg	5 mg IR BID or 10 mg ER QAM
Focalin 5 mg BID	10 mg IR BID
Focalin XR 10 mg QAM	20 mg IR QAM
Jornay PM 20 mg QPM	4 mg IR TID
Jornay PM 100 mg QPM	20 mg IR TID
Quillichew ER 20 mg QAM	10 mg IR BID or 20 mg ER QAM
Quillichew ER 30 mg QAM	15 mg IR BID or 30 mg ER QAM
Quillichew ER 40 mg QAM	20 mg IR BID or 40 mg ER QAM
Quillivant XR 10 mg (2 mL) QAM	5 mg IR BID or 10 mg ER QAM
Quillivant XR 20 mg (4 mL) QAM	10 mg IR BID or 20 mg ER QAM
Quillivant XR 30 mg (6 mL) QAM	15 mg IR BID or 30 mg ER QAM
Quillivant XR 40 mg (8 mL) QAM	20 mg IR BID or 40 mg ER QAM
Amphetamines	
Alternative Formulation	**Regular Mixed Amphetamine Salts Equivalent**
Adzenys XR ODT 3.1 mg QAM	2.5 mg IR BID or 5 mg ER QAM
Adzenys XR ODT 6.3 mg QAM	5 mg IR BID or 10 mg ER QAM
Adzenys XR ODT 9.4 mg QAM	7.5 mg IR BID or 15 mg ER QAM
Adzenys XR ODT 12.5 mg QAM	10 mg IR BID or 20 mg ER QAM
Adzenys XR ODT 15.7 mg QAM	12.5 mg IR BID or 25 mg ER QAM
Adzenys XR ODT 18.8 mg QAM	15 mg IR BID or 30 mg ER QAM
Adzenys ER 3.125 mg (2.5 mL) QAM	2.5 mg IR BID or 5 mg ER QAM
Adzenys ER 6.25 mg (5 mL) QAM	5 mg IR BID or 10 mg ER QAM
Adzenys ER 9.375 mg (7.5 mL) QAM	7.5 mg IR BID or 15 mg ER QAM
Adzenys ER 12.5 mg (10 mL) QAM	10 mg IR BID or 20 mg ER QAM
Adzenys ER 15.625 mg (12.5 mL) QAM	12.5 mg IR BID or 25 mg ER QAM
Adzenys ER 18.75 mg (15 mL) QAM	15 mg IR BID or 30 mg ER QAM
Dyanavel XR 6.25 mg (2.5 mL)	5 mg IR BID or 10 mg ER QAM
Dyanavel XR 12.5 mg (5 mL)	10 mg IR BID or 20 mg ER QAM
Dyanavel XR 18.75 mg (7.5 mL)	15 mg IR BID or 30 mg ER QAM
Mydayis 25 mg QAM	20 mg ER QAM
Vyvanse 30 mg QAM	5 mg IR BID or 10 mg ER QAM
Vyvanse 50 mg QAM	10 mg IR BID or 20 mg ER QAM
Vyvanse 70 mg QAM	15 mg IR BID or 30 mg ER QAM

IR = immediate release; ER = extended release

[1]These are approximate equivalencies provided as guidance; taper and titrate each agent based on recommended dosing when switching, or start the new stimulant at a somewhat lower dose than the calculation

AMPHETAMINE (Adzenys XR-ODT, Dyanavel XR, Evekeo) Fact Sheet [G]

BOTTOM LINE:
Newer formulations of an old drug come with a high price tag. Stick to the usual amphetamine products like mixed amphetamine salts unless liquid or ODT dosing is absolutely necessary.

PEDIATRIC FDA INDICATIONS:
ADHD (Adzenys XR-ODT and Dyanavel XR: children >6; Evekeo: children >3).

ADULT FDA INDICATIONS:
ADHD (Adzenys XR-ODT); narcolepsy (Evekeo); obesity (Evekeo).

OFF-LABEL USES:
Treatment-resistant depression.

DOSAGE FORMS:
- **Tablets (Evekeo, [G]):** 5 mg, 10 mg (scored); **(Evekeo ODT):** 2.5 mg, 5 mg, 10 mg, 15 mg, 20 mg.
- **ER tablets (Dyanavel XR):** 5 mg (scored), 10 mg, 15 mg, 20 mg.
- **ER orally disintegrating tablets (Adzenys XR-ODT):** 3.1 mg, 6.3 mg, 9.4 mg, 12.5 mg, 15.7 mg, 18.8 mg.
- **ER oral suspension (Dyanavel XR):** 2.5 mg/mL; **(Adzenys ER):** 1.25 mg/mL.

PEDIATRIC DOSAGE GUIDANCE:
- Tablets (Evekeo, [G]):
  - Children 3–5: Start 2.5 mg QAM, increase in 2.5 mg/day increments weekly to maximum of 40 mg/day in divided doses.
  - Children 6–17: Start 5 mg QAM, increase in 5 mg/day increments weekly to maximum of 40 mg/day in divided doses.
- ER ODT (Adzenys XR-ODT) or Adzenys ER oral suspension:
  - Start 6.3 mg QAM, increase in 3.1 mg (2.5 mL)/day–6.3 mg (5 mL)/day increments weekly. Maximum of 18.8 mg (15 mL)/day (ages 6–12) or 12.5 mg (10 mL)/day (ages 13–17).
- ER oral suspension (Dyanavel XR):
  - Start 2.5–5 mg QAM, increase in 2.5–10 mg/day increments every four to seven days. Maximum 20 mg/day.

MONITORING: Weight, height, BP/P; ECG.

COST: [G]: $$$; others: $$$$

SIDE EFFECTS:
- Most common: Abdominal pain, decreased appetite, weight loss, insomnia, headache, nervousness.
- Serious but rare: See class warnings in chapter introduction.

MECHANISM, PHARMACOKINETICS, AND DRUG INTERACTIONS:
- Stimulant that inhibits reuptake of dopamine and norepinephrine.
- Metabolized primarily via CYP2D6; t ½: 11 hours.
- Avoid use with MAOIs, antacids.

EVIDENCE AND CLINICAL PEARLS:
- FDA approved, many studies, history of clinical efficacy and safety, and larger effect size than non-stimulants.
- Racemic l-isomer is more potent than d-isomer in peripheral activity (more cardiovascular effects, tics).
- There may be less appetite suppressant effects with racemic mixture compared to dextroamphetamine.
- Divide IR (Evekeo) doses by intervals of four to six hours.
- Approximate equivalence doses of Adzenys XR-ODT and mixed amphetamine salts XR (Adderall XR) are: 3.1 mg = 5 mg, 6.3 mg = 10 mg, 9.4 mg = 15 mg, 12.5 mg = 20 mg, 15.7 mg = 25 mg, 18.8 mg = 30 mg.
- Shake Dyanavel XR oral suspension for extended release. 2.5 mg/mL = 4 mg of mixed amphetamine salts.
- Amphetamines are not interchangeable on a mg:mg basis. When switching, use a lowered dose and adjust.

FUN FACT:
The term "amphetamine" is the contracted form of the chemical "alpha-methylphenethylamine." Its first pharmacologic use was when pharmaceutical company Smith, Kline and French sold amphetamine under the trade name Benzedrine as a decongestant inhaler.

ATOMOXETINE (Strattera) Fact Sheet [G]

BOTTOM LINE:
Advantages: Unlike stimulants, atomoxetine has no abuse potential, causes less insomnia and anxiety, and is unlikely to worsen tics.
Disadvantages: It is generally less effective than stimulants, and takes longer to work (two to four weeks).

PEDIATRIC FDA INDICATIONS:
ADHD (6–17 years).

ADULT FDA INDICATIONS:
ADHD.

OFF-LABEL USES:
Treatment-resistant depression.

DOSAGE FORMS:
Capsules (G): 10 mg, 18 mg, 25 mg, 40 mg, 60 mg, 80 mg, 100 mg.

PEDIATRIC DOSAGE GUIDANCE:
- Children >70 kg: Start 40 mg QAM for three days, ↑ to 80 mg QAM, may ↑ to 100 mg/day after two to four weeks if needed (max 100 mg/day); may divide doses >40 mg/day (divided dosing in morning and late afternoon/early evening).
- Children <70 kg: Start 0.5 mg/kg QAM for three days, ↑ to 1.2 mg/kg QAM, may ↑ to max 1.4 mg/kg/day or 100 mg/day (whichever is less) after two to four weeks, if needed; may divide doses >0.5 mg/kg/day (divided dosing in morning and late afternoon/early evening).

MONITORING: BP/P, LFTs.

COST: $

SIDE EFFECTS:
- Most common: Headache, abdominal pain, decreased appetite, fatigue, nausea, vomiting.
- Serious but rare: Class warning for suicidal ideation in children and teens. Severe hepatic injury including increased hepatic enzymes (up to 40 times normal) and jaundice (bilirubin up to 12 times upper limit of normal). Increased blood pressure (↑ 15–20 mmHg) and heart rate (↑ 20 bpm).

MECHANISM, PHARMACOKINETICS, AND DRUG INTERACTIONS:
- Selective norepinephrine reuptake inhibitor (NRI).
- Metabolized primarily via CYP2D6; t ½: 5 hours.
- Avoid use with MAOIs. Exercise caution with 2D6 inhibitors such as fluoxetine, paroxetine, and quinidine (increased atomoxetine serum levels); use slower titration and do not exceed 80 mg/day in presence of 2D6 inhibitors or in 2D6 poor metabolizers.

EVIDENCE AND CLINICAL PEARLS:
- Effective and FDA approved for ADHD; however, several studies clearly show it does not produce as robust of a treatment effect as stimulants.
- QAM dosing is as effective as BID, but BID dosing has better GI tolerability. Can also be dosed at bedtime if it causes fatigue.
- Appears to be more effective in improving attention than in controlling hyperactivity.
- Of the two NRIs available for ADHD, atomoxetine is cheaper than viloxazine.

FUN FACT:
Atomoxetine was originally known as "tomoxetine"; however, the FDA requested that the name be changed because the similarity to "tamoxifen" could lead to dispensing errors.

CLONIDINE (Catapres, Kapvay) Fact Sheet [G]

BOTTOM LINE:
Clonidine is a good option in kids with ADHD who also have tics, who experience excessive anxiety or insomnia on stimulants, or in whom substance misuse is a concern. Its delayed onset of effect (two to four weeks) and lower efficacy rates make it a second-line choice for ADHD generally; however, it can also be used as an add-on to stimulant medication. Commonly used off label for anxiety and insomnia, but efficacy data are limited.

PEDIATRIC FDA INDICATIONS:
ADHD (6–17 years [ER formulation only]).

ADULT FDA INDICATIONS:
Hypertension.

OFF-LABEL USES:
ADHD (IR); insomnia; anxiety; PTSD; opioid withdrawal; autism; ODD; Tourette's and motor tics; migraine prophylaxis; aggression.

DOSAGE FORMS:
• **IR tablets (Catapres, [G]):** 0.1 mg, 0.2 mg, 0.3 mg.
• **ER tablets (Kapvay, [G]):** 0.1 mg, 0.2 mg.
• **Patch (Catapres-TTS, [G]):** 0.1 mg/day, 0.2 mg/day, 0.3 mg/day.

PEDIATRIC DOSAGE GUIDANCE:
• ADHD or anxiety:
  – ER: 0.1 mg QHS; increase by 0.1 mg/day weekly and give divided BID; max 0.4 mg QD.
  – IR: 0.05 mg QHS; increase by 0.05 mg/day increments every three to seven days; max 0.2 mg/day for 27–40.5 kg, 0.3 mg/day for 40.5–45 kg, or 0.4 mg/day for >45 kg; doses may be divided up to QID dosing.
• Insomnia: Start 0.05 mg IR QHS, titrate if needed by 0.05 mg (<45 kg) or 0.1 mg (>45 kg) increments every three to seven days; max 0.4 mg nightly, though most will respond to doses ≤0.2 mg at bedtime.

MONITORING: BP.

COST: $

SIDE EFFECTS:
• Most common: Somnolence, fatigue, dizziness, headache.
• Serious but rare: Hypotension, syncope, orthostasis.

MECHANISM, PHARMACOKINETICS, AND DRUG INTERACTIONS:
• Centrally acting alpha-2 adrenergic agonist.
• Metabolized primary through CYP2D6; t ½: 12–16 hours.
• Avoid use with MAOIs. Additive effects with other antihypertensives. Caution with 2D6 inhibitors (eg, paroxetine, fluoxetine, duloxetine).

EVIDENCE AND CLINICAL PEARLS:
• Studies support the use of clonidine to decrease residual hyperactivity, impulsivity, and aggression in ADHD.
• Several small limited (chart review, case series, descriptive, or retrospective) studies have supported the efficacy of clonidine as a sleep aid in autistic kids as well as children with and without ADHD, developmental delays, and genetic syndromes; however, a small systematic chart review showed significant subjective improvement in sleep in children, but only a nonsignificant trend for improvement of sleep in adolescents.
• Avoid abrupt discontinuation because of potential risk for rebound hypertension. When discontinuing, taper in no more than 0.1 mg/day decrements every three to seven days to reduce the risk of rebound hypertension. If a child misses two or more consecutive doses, consider repeating titration.
• Although a few studies support use of the patch for treating tic disorders, the patch formulation is not typically used except for treating hypertension because its effects on BP may be prolonged and continue even after patch removal.
• Many child psychiatrists prefer clonidine as an agent for sleep, but little empirical evidence exists to support this use. Still, anecdotal clinical experience suggests clonidine is generally safe and effective for insomnia, particularly in kids with ADHD.
• Generally more sedating than guanfacine.

FUN FACT:
In the early 1960s, Boehringer Ingelheim wished to synthesize a peripherally active adrenergic drug for nasal decongestion as nose drops. After administering the potential compound to a secretary, she fell asleep for 24 hours, developing low blood pressure, low pulse, and dry mouth. This compound was subsequently developed as clonidine for treating hypertension.

DEXMETHYLPHENIDATE (Azstarys, Focalin, Focalin XR) Fact Sheet [G]

BOTTOM LINE:
Focalin is just Ritalin but more potent. It's available as a generic and may mean fewer tablets for patients. Focalin XR only recently went generic. Azstarys is a newly approved (and expensive) combination of Focalin and a prodrug version of Focalin—the Focalin is absorbed quickly while the prodrug is absorbed more slowly (it's the Vyvanse of methylphenidate, with less potential misuse than Focalin).

PEDIATRIC FDA INDICATIONS:
ADHD (6–17 years).

ADULT FDA INDICATIONS:
ADHD (Azstarys, Focalin XR).

OFF-LABEL USES:
Narcolepsy; obesity; treatment-resistant depression.

DOSAGE FORMS:
- **Dexmethylphenidate tablets (Focalin, [G]):** 2.5 mg, 5 mg, 10 mg.
- **Dexmethylphenidate ER capsules (Focalin XR, [G]):** 5 mg, 10 mg, 15 mg, 20 mg, 25 mg, 30 mg, 35 mg, 40 mg.
- **Serdexmethylphenidate/dexmethylphenidate ER capsules (Azstarys):** 26.1/5.2 mg, 39.2/7.8 mg, 52.3/10.4 mg.

PEDIATRIC DOSAGE GUIDANCE:
- d-MPH IR: Start 2.5 mg BID, ↑ by 5–10 mg/day every seven days. Max 20 mg/day; divide IR doses by at least four hours.
- d-MPH ER: Start 5 mg QAM, ↑ by 5 mg/day every seven days. Max 30 mg/day.
- Serdex-MPH/d-MPH: Start 39.2/7.8 mg QAM, ↑ to max dose of 52.3/10.4 mg after one week if indicated.

MONITORING: Weight, height, BP/P; ECG.

COST: IR: $; ER: $$; Azstarys: $$$$

SIDE EFFECTS:
- Most common: Decreased appetite, insomnia, anxiety, GI distress, irritability, tics, headache, tachycardia, hypertension, dry mouth.
- Serious but rare: See cardiovascular class warning in chapter introduction.

MECHANISM, PHARMACOKINETICS, AND DRUG INTERACTIONS:
- Stimulant that inhibits reuptake of dopamine and norepinephrine.
- Serdexmethylphenidate (Serdex-MPH) is a prodrug of dexmethylphenidate (d-MPH). d-MPH is metabolized primarily via de-esterification, not CYP450; t ½: 2–4.5 hours (2–3 hours in children); d-MPH ER delivers 50% of dose immediately and 50% about five hours later. Azstarys t ½: 6–12 hours; delivers 30% d-MPH immediately and 70% as prodrug.
- Avoid use with MAOIs.

EVIDENCE AND CLINICAL PEARLS:
- Several randomized controlled trials and meta-analyses have shown dexmethylphenidate, like other stimulants, is effective for ADHD with a large treatment effect size.
- Focalin is the d-isomer of methylphenidate and is twice as potent as methylphenidate, which is why it is prescribed at about half the dose. Serdex-MPH is a prodrug, converted to d-MPH in the lower GI tract.
- Use the same total daily dose of Focalin IR as Focalin XR. The combined dose of Azstarys 26.1/5.2, 39.2/7.8, or 52.3/10.4 mg is equivalent to 20, 30, or 40 mg of Focalin, respectively.
- Focalin XR capsules contain two kinds of beads: Half are immediate-release beads and half are enteric-coated delayed-release beads. A single, once-daily dose of XR capsule provides the same amount of dexmethylphenidate as two IR tablets given four hours apart.
- The ER capsules cannot be split in half. However, they can be opened and the beads sprinkled over food. The patient should then eat all that food—eating half won't work to split the dose accurately because it won't be possible to determine if the eaten portion contains more immediate-release or delayed-release beads.
- Give with food if GI side effects occur.

FUN FACT:
With two stereoactive centers, methylphenidate has four possible stereoisomers. Of the four, dexmethylphenidate is the most active biologically.

DEXTROAMPHETAMINE (Dexedrine, ProCentra, Zenzedi) Fact Sheet [G]

BOTTOM LINE:
Good drug with very long history of experience, available in short- and long-acting formulations as generics.

PEDIATRIC FDA INDICATIONS:
ADHD (3–17 years); **narcolepsy** (6–17 years).

ADULT FDA INDICATIONS:
Narcolepsy.

OFF-LABEL USES:
Obesity; treatment-resistant depression.

DOSAGE FORMS:
- **Tablets (Dexedrine, [G]):** 5 mg, 10 mg (scored).
- **Tablets (Zenzedi):** 2.5 mg, 5 mg, 7.5 mg, 10 mg, 15 mg, 20 mg, 30 mg (5 mg scored, 10 mg double scored; rest unscored).
- **ER capsules (Dexedrine Spansules, [G]):** 5 mg, 10 mg, 15 mg.
- **Liquid (ProCentra, [G]):** 5 mg/5 mL.

PEDIATRIC DOSAGE GUIDANCE:
- ADHD (IR and ER):
  - Children >6 years: Start 5 mg QAM; ↑ by 5 mg/day at weekly intervals to max 60 mg/day, though doses >40 mg/day rarely more effective. Divide IR dose QD–TID.
  - Children 3–5 years: Start 2.5 mg QAM; ↑ by 2.5 mg/day weekly to max 60 mg/day, though doses >40 mg/day rarely more effective. Divide IR dose QD–TID.
- Narcolepsy (IR and ER):
  - Start 5 mg QAM (ages 6–11) or 10 mg QAM (ages 12–17); ↑ by 5 mg/day (ages 6–11) or 10 mg/day (ages 12–17) weekly to max 60 mg/day. Divide IR dose QD–TID.

MONITORING: Weight, height, BP/P; ECG.

COST: IR/ER: $ (ProCentra: $$$)

SIDE EFFECTS:
- Most common: Abdominal pain, anorexia, nausea, tics, insomnia, tachycardia, headache.
- Serious but rare: See class warnings in chapter introduction.

MECHANISM, PHARMACOKINETICS, AND DRUG INTERACTIONS:
- Stimulant that inhibits reuptake of dopamine and norepinephrine.
- Metabolized primarily through CYP450 2D6 (minor) and glucuronidation; t ½: 12 hours.
- Avoid use with MAOIs, antacids.

EVIDENCE AND CLINICAL PEARLS:
- At least five randomized clinical trials, some dating back to the 1970s, support the efficacy of dextroamphetamine in children with ADHD.
- Dextroamphetamine is the more potent d-isomer of amphetamine; it has potentially less peripheral effects (eg, motor tics) than racemic mix (eg, mixed amphetamine salts like Adderall, amphetamine, or methamphetamine).
- Doses of IR tablets and oral solution can be given at intervals of four to six hours.
- Dextroamphetamine is the only stimulant, other than Adderall IR, approved for children <6 years (approved for children >3 years).
- The newer Zenzedi brand offers more dosing flexibility options, but is more expensive than generic IR tablets.
- Available in a new patch formulation as Xelstrym (see fact sheet).
- Also available as D,L racemic mixture of amphetamine as Evekeo tablets, Adzenys XR-ODT, and Dyanavel XR oral suspension (see amphetamine fact sheet).

FUN FACT:
Dexys Midnight Runners, the British band famous for its song "Come On Eileen" (1982), derived their name from Dexedrine—"Dexys" after the drug's name and "Midnight Runners" in reference to the energy it provides.

DEXTROAMPHETAMINE TRANSDERMAL (Xelstrym) Fact Sheet

BOTTOM LINE:
A patch option in the amphetamine class of stimulants for kids who cannot use the wide array of oral stimulants available today. Minimal data and less experience than with methylphenidate transdermal (Daytrana), but similar to Daytrana in terms of high cost, lag time for onset of effect, and side effects.

PEDIATRIC FDA INDICATIONS:
ADHD (6–17 years).

ADULT FDA INDICATIONS:
ADHD.

DOSAGE FORMS:
Transdermal patch: 4.5 mg, 9 mg, 13.5 mg, 18 mg/9 hour.

PEDIATRIC DOSAGE GUIDANCE:
Start 4.5 mg/9 hour patch QAM (for initial therapy or for patients switching from other amphetamine preparations, regardless of dose). Apply to hip, upper arm, chest, upper back, or flank two hours before an effect is needed and remove nine hours after application (drug effects may persist for five hours after removal). Increase dose at weekly intervals by using next-higher-dose system. May be removed in <9 hours if shorter duration is desired or if late-day side effects occur. Rotate application sites. Max 18 mg QD.

MONITORING: Weight, height, BP/P; ECG.

COST: $$$$

SIDE EFFECTS:
- Most common: Decreased appetite, headache, insomnia, tic, abdominal pain, vomiting, nausea, irritability, increased BP and pulse. Application site reactions and sensitization may occur.
- Serious but rare: See class warnings in chapter introduction.

MECHANISM, PHARMACOKINETICS, AND DRUG INTERACTIONS:
- Stimulant that inhibits reuptake of dopamine and norepinephrine.
- Metabolized primarily through CYP450 2D6 (minor) and glucuronidation; t ½: 6.4 hours (11.5 hours in adults).
- Avoid use with MAOIs, antacids.

EVIDENCE AND CLINICAL PEARLS:
- Approval was based on a two-week, randomized, double-blind, placebo-controlled, crossover, modified-analog classroom study in 110 pediatric patients with ADHD ages 6–17. Efficacy measure assessed was the Swanson, Kotkin, Angler, M. Flynn, and Pelham (SKAMP) score, a scale specific to the classroom setting.
- Dextroamphetamine is the more potent d-isomer of amphetamine; it has potentially less peripheral effects (eg, motor tics) than racemic mix (eg, mixed amphetamine salts like Adderall, amphetamine, or methamphetamine).
- The manufacturer, Noven Pharmaceuticals, Inc. recommends against cutting the patch (eg to adjust the dosage).

FUN FACT:
While Daytrana is approved for pediatric use only, Xelstrym is also approved for use in adults.

GUANFACINE (Intuniv, Tenex) Fact Sheet [G]

BOTTOM LINE:
Guanfacine's advantages over stimulants include no worsening of tic disorders, lack of misuse potential, and no insomnia. It can also be used as an add-on to stimulant medication. However, its delayed onset of effect (two to four weeks) and lower efficacy rates make it a second-line choice for ADHD generally. ER is now available in generic and easier to use than IR. Commonly used off label for anxiety and insomnia, but efficacy data are limited.

PEDIATRIC FDA INDICATIONS:
ADHD (6–17 years [ER formulation only]), as monotherapy or adjunctive therapy to stimulants.

ADULT FDA INDICATIONS:
Hypertension.

OFF-LABEL USES:
Conduct disorder; Tourette's and motor tics; agitation in autistic kids; migraine prophylaxis; opioid withdrawal; anxiety and PTSD; insomnia.

DOSAGE FORMS:
- **IR tablets (Tenex, [G]):** 1 mg, 2 mg.
- **ER tablets (Intuniv, [G]):** 1 mg, 2 mg, 3 mg, 4 mg.

PEDIATRIC DOSAGE GUIDANCE:
- ADHD or anxiety:
  - IR dosing depends on weight:
    - 27–40.5 kg (55–90 lbs): Start 0.5 mg QHS, ↑ by 0.5 mg/day at weekly intervals up to 1.5 mg/day; may ↑ to 2 mg/day after two weeks; max 2 mg/day in two to four divided doses.
    - 40.5–45 kg (90–99 lbs): Start 0.5 mg QHS, ↑ by 0.5 mg/day at weekly intervals; max 1 mg per dose, 3 mg/day.
    - >45 kg (>99 lbs): Start 1 mg QHS, ↑ by 1 mg/day at weekly intervals up to 3 mg/day; may ↑ to 4 mg/day after two weeks; max 1 mg per dose, 4 mg/day.
  - ER: Start 1 mg QHS, ↑ by 1 mg/day at weekly intervals; max 4 mg/day. Alternative: 0.05–0.12 mg/kg QD or QHS; max 4 mg/day. Doses up to 7 mg/day ER studied as monotherapy in adolescents.
- Insomnia: Use IR: Start low, go slow, typically 0.5 mg QHS, increasing by 0.5 mg/day at weekly intervals; max 3 mg/day.

MONITORING: BP.

COST: $

SIDE EFFECTS:
- Most common: Dry mouth, somnolence, dizziness, constipation, fatigue, headache.
- Serious but rare: Hypotension, syncope, orthostasis.

MECHANISM, PHARMACOKINETICS, AND DRUG INTERACTIONS:
- Centrally acting, selective alpha-2 adrenergic agonist.
- Metabolized primarily through CYP3A4; t ½: 13–14 hours in children (16–18 hours in adults).
- Avoid use with MAOIs. Caution with 3A4 inhibitors (eg, clarithromycin, fluvoxamine) and inducers (eg, St. John's wort, carbamazepine).

EVIDENCE AND CLINICAL PEARLS:
- At least six randomized placebo-controlled trials and a meta-analysis show efficacy in children with ADHD.
- A pilot study of 83 children with GAD, separation anxiety, or social anxiety found guanfacine treatment resulted in greater subjective improvement of anxiety than placebo, but no improvement on other measures of anxiety.
- One negative randomized trial for insomnia in children with ADHD found decreased total sleep time of nearly an hour, with kids taking more time to fall asleep.
- Guanfacine IR and ER are not interchangeable on a mg:mg basis. When switching, taper and retitrate.
- Guanfacine tends to be less sedating than clonidine, another alpha-agonist.
- ER tablets should not be taken with a high-fat meal due to increased medication exposure.
- Minimize side effects, especially somnolence, by administering at bedtime.
- Monitor BP, especially during initial dosing titration.
- There is a risk of nervousness, anxiety, and possibly rebound hypertension two to four days after abrupt discontinuation. Taper dose in 1 mg/day decrements every three to seven days.
- If a child misses two or more consecutive doses, consider repeating titration.

FUN FACT:
Some prescribers have taken advantage of guanfacine's sympatholytic properties for the treatment of anxiety disorders in children as well as nightmares and dissociative symptoms in PTSD.

LISDEXAMFETAMINE (Vyvanse) Fact Sheet

BOTTOM LINE:
Vyvanse may have a gentler, "smoother" side effect profile than other amphetamines, and probably has a lower risk of diversion or misuse. However, its high cost means insurance companies don't like to pay for it without prior authorizations.

PEDIATRIC FDA INDICATIONS:
ADHD (6–17 years).

ADULT FDA INDICATIONS:
ADHD; binge eating disorder (BED).

OFF-LABEL USES:
Narcolepsy; obesity; treatment-resistant depression.

DOSAGE FORMS:
- **Capsules:** 10 mg, 20 mg, 30 mg, 40 mg, 50 mg, 60 mg, 70 mg.
- **Chewable tablets:** 10 mg, 20 mg, 30 mg, 40 mg, 50 mg, 60 mg.

PEDIATRIC DOSAGE GUIDANCE:
Start 30 mg QAM, ↑ by 10–20 mg/day at weekly intervals. Target lowest effective dose; max 70 mg/day.

MONITORING: Weight, height, BP/P; ECG.

COST: $$$$

SIDE EFFECTS:
- Most common: Insomnia, anorexia, abdominal pain, irritability, agitation, tics, decreased appetite, increased heart rate, jitteriness, anxiety.
- Serious but rare: See class warnings in chapter introduction.

MECHANISM, PHARMACOKINETICS, AND DRUG INTERACTIONS:
- Stimulant that inhibits reuptake of dopamine and norepinephrine.
- Metabolized primarily through non-CYP-mediated hepatic and/or intestinal metabolism; t ½: lisdexamfetamine (inactive prodrug) <1 hour; dextroamphetamine (active metabolite) 12 hours. Dextroamphetamine metabolized by CYP2D6.
- Avoid use with MAOIs and antacids. Caution with antihypertensives (decreased efficacy of antihypertensive). Caution with 2D6 inhibitors, which may increase stimulant effects.

EVIDENCE AND CLINICAL PEARLS:
- At least five randomized controlled trials and a meta-analysis support efficacy of lisdexamfetamine in children with ADHD.
- Lisdexamfetamine is dextroamphetamine with the chemical lysine bound to it, which renders it inactive. It remains inactive until GI enzymes cleave off lysine and convert it to active dextroamphetamine. This means that people who misuse it can't get high by snorting it or injecting it.
- Anecdotally, Vyvanse has a more gradual onset and offset than other stimulants, and may cause fewer side effects than other amphetamines.
- Taking with food decreases the effect slightly and delays peak levels by an hour. If patients feel it's not "kicking in" fast enough, have them take it earlier or on an empty stomach.
- Lisdexamfetamine 70 mg is equivalent to 30 mg of mixed amphetamine salts (Adderall).
- While indicated for BED, it is not approved for use as a weight-loss or anti-obesity agent, nor has it been studied in children.

FUN FACT:
The manufacturer of Vyvanse pursued an indication as an add-on medication for depression, but disappointing results in clinical trials put an end to this effort.

METHAMPHETAMINE (Desoxyn) Fact Sheet [G]

BOTTOM LINE:
Highly addictive substance; its use is generally not recommended. Watch the television show *Breaking Bad* if you're not convinced!

PEDIATRIC FDA INDICATIONS:
ADHD (6–17 years); **obesity** (12–17 years).

ADULT FDA INDICATIONS:
Obesity.

DOSAGE FORMS:
Tablets (G): 5 mg.

PEDIATRIC DOSAGE GUIDANCE:
ADHD: Start 5 mg QAM–BID, ↑ by 5 mg/day at weekly intervals to max 20 mg/day, divided BID.

MONITORING: Weight, height, BP/P; ECG.

COST: $$$$

SIDE EFFECTS:
- Most common: Anorexia, tachycardia, dizziness, insomnia, tremor, tics, restlessness, headache, constipation (decreased GI motility). Dental complications, such as poor dental hygiene, diffuse cavities, bruxism, and tooth wear, may develop with misuse.
- Serious but rare: See class warnings in chapter introduction.

MECHANISM, PHARMACOKINETICS, AND DRUG INTERACTIONS:
- Stimulant that inhibits reuptake of dopamine and norepinephrine.
- Metabolized primarily through CYP2D6 to active metabolite (amphetamine); t ½: 4–5 hours.
- Avoid use with MAOIs and antacids. Caution with 2D6 inhibitors, which may increase stimulant effects.

EVIDENCE AND CLINICAL PEARLS:
- FDA indication, but very limited published data in children.
- High risk of misuse.
- Not widely used (DEA reports that there were only 16,000 prescriptions written in 2012). When prescribed for obesity, the recommendation is for short-term (ie, a few weeks) use only and as an adjunct to caloric restriction due to its high addiction and diversion potential.
- CNS stimulating effect is approximately equal to or greater than that of amphetamine but less than that of dextroamphetamine; less BP elevation than with amphetamine.

FUN FACTS:
Desoxyn is the same as the abused street drug methamphetamine, just pharmaceutical grade. Although methamphetamine and amphetamine were long thought to be available only via laboratories, methamphetamine has been reported to occur naturally in certain acacia trees that grow in West Texas.

METHYLPHENIDATE IR (Methylin, Ritalin) Fact Sheet [G]

BOTTOM LINE:
Better side effect profile and somewhat lower misuse potential than amphetamines. However, patients often prefer the "kick" they get from Adderall.

PEDIATRIC FDA INDICATIONS:
ADHD (6–17 years).

ADULT FDA INDICATIONS:
ADHD; narcolepsy.

OFF-LABEL USES:
Obesity; treatment-resistant depression.

DOSAGE FORMS:
• **Tablets (Ritalin, [G]):** 5 mg, 10 mg, 20 mg.
• **Chewable tablets (Methylin CT, [G]):** 2.5 mg, 5 mg, 10 mg.
• **Oral solution (Methylin, [G]):** 5 mg/5 mL, 10 mg/5 mL.

PEDIATRIC DOSAGE GUIDANCE:
• ADHD: Children 6–17 years: Start 0.3 mg/kg BID or 2.5–5 mg BID before breakfast and lunch, increase by 0.1 mg/kg/dose or 5–10 mg/day at weekly intervals to a max of 2 mg/kg/day or 60 mg/day.
• Narcolepsy: Same dosing as ADHD.

MONITORING: Weight, height, BP/P; ECG.

COST: $; chewable tablets: $$$

SIDE EFFECTS:
• Most common: Insomnia, headache, nervousness, abdominal pain, nausea, vomiting, anorexia, weight loss, affect lability, tics.
• Serious but rare: See class warnings in chapter introduction.

MECHANISM, PHARMACOKINETICS, AND DRUG INTERACTIONS:
• Stimulant that inhibits reuptake of dopamine and norepinephrine.
• Hepatic metabolism via carboxylesterase CES1A1, not CYP450 isoenzymes; t ½: 2–4 hours.
• Avoid use with MAOIs, antacids.

EVIDENCE AND CLINICAL PEARLS:
• FDA approved with many studies and long history of clinical use supporting its efficacy and safety, with a larger treatment effect size than non-stimulant medications.
• Methylphenidate generally causes fewer side effects than amphetamine preparations—patients are less likely to report feeling "wired."
• While all stimulants may unmask tics, a Cochrane review of eight randomized trials showed that methylphenidate did not worsen tics in children with ADHD and a tic disorder; in some cases it even improved tics.
• Methylin chewable tablet: Administer with at least 8 ounces of water or other fluid.

FUN FACT:
Methylphenidate was synthesized by Ciba (now Novartis) chemist Leandro Panizzon. His wife, Marguerite, had low blood pressure and would take the stimulant before playing tennis. He named the substance "Ritaline" (yes, with the "e" on the end) after his wife's nickname, Rita.

METHYLPHENIDATE ER (Concerta, Ritalin SR and LA, others) Fact Sheet [G]

BOTTOM LINE:
There are many longer-acting methylphenidate preparations. Two good options are Concerta and Ritalin LA, available as generics.

PEDIATRIC FDA INDICATIONS:
ADHD (6–17 years).

ADULT FDA INDICATIONS:
ADHD; narcolepsy.

OFF-LABEL USES:
Obesity; treatment-resistant depression.

DOSAGE FORMS (more commonly used):
- Tablets
  - **SR tablets (Ritalin SR, Metadate ER, Methylin ER, [G]):** 10 mg, 20 mg.
  - **ER capsule osmotic release oral system (OROS) (Concerta, [G]):** 18 mg, 27 mg, 36 mg, 54 mg (22% IR/78% ER).
- Capsules
  - **Ritalin LA, [G]:** 10 mg, 20 mg, 30 mg, 40 mg, 60 mg (50% IR/50% ER).
  - **Metadate CD, [G]:** 10 mg, 20 mg, 30 mg, 40 mg, 50 mg, 60 mg (30% IR/70% ER).
  - **Aptensio XR:** 10 mg, 15 mg, 20 mg, 30 mg, 40 mg, 50 mg, 60 mg (40% IR/60% ER).
  - **Adhansia XR:** 25 mg, 35 mg, 45 mg, 55 mg, 70 mg, 85 mg (20% IR/80% ER)
  - **Jornay PM:** 20 mg, 40 mg, 60 mg, 80 mg, 100 mg (onset delayed 10 hours).
  - **ER oral suspension (Quillivant XR):** 25 mg/5 mL (20% IR/80% ER).
  - **ER chewable tablets (Quillichew ER):** 20 mg, 30 mg (scored), 40 mg (scored) (30% IR/70% ER).
  - **ER orally disintegrating tablets (Cotempla XR-ODT):** 8.6 mg, 17.3 mg, 25.9 mg (25% IR/75% ER).

PEDIATRIC DOSAGE GUIDANCE:
- Intermediate-acting (Ritalin SR, Metadate ER, Methylin ER): Titrate to effective daily dose with IR, then switch to equivalent eight-hour SR or ER dose QAM–BID or start 10 mg QAM and increase by 10 mg/day increments weekly; max 60 mg/day.
- Long-acting (Aptensio XR, Metadate CD, Ritalin LA, Quillivant XR, Quillichew ER): Start 10–20 mg QAM; ↑ by 10 mg/day at weekly intervals; max 60 mg/day.
- Long-acting (Adhansia XR): Start 25 mg QAM; ↑ by 10–15 mg/day at weekly intervals; max 70 mg/day (children) and 85 mg/day (adults).
- Long-acting (Cotempla XR-ODT):
  - Start 17.3 mg QAM; ↑ by 8.6–17.3 mg/day at weekly intervals; max 51.8 mg/day.
  - 8.6 mg, 17.3 mg, 25.9 mg equivalent to 10 mg, 20 mg, 30 mg of other methylphenidate formulations, respectively.
- Long-acting (Concerta):
  - Start 18 mg QAM (ages 6–12) or 36 mg (ages 13–17) QAM; ↑ by 18 mg/day in weekly intervals to max 54 mg/day (ages 6–12) or 72 mg/day (ages 13–17).
  - If switching from different form of methylphenidate:
    - 10–15 mg/day: Use 18 mg QAM.
    - 20–30 mg/day: Use 36 mg QAM.
    - 30–45 mg/day: Use 54 mg QAM.
    - 40–60 mg/day: Use 72 mg QAM.
    - 27 mg dose is available for situations in which a dose between 18 mg and 36 mg is desired.
- Jornay PM: Start 20 mg daily in the evening and increase in increments of 20 mg/day up to maximum of 100 mg/day. Adjust timing between 6:30 and 9:30 p.m.

COST: $$; Aptensio XR, Cotempla XR-ODT, Concerta, Jornay PM, Quillivant XR, and Quillichew ER: $$$$

SIDE EFFECTS AND MECHANISM, MONITORING, PHARMACOKINETICS, AND DRUG INTERACTIONS:
Weight, height, BP/P; ECG. See methylphenidate IR fact sheet.

EVIDENCE AND CLINICAL PEARLS:
- FDA approved with many studies and long history of clinical use supporting its efficacy and safety, with a larger treatment effect size than non-stimulant medications.
- ER capsules contain mixture of 30% IR and 70% ER beads. Aptensio XR, a new branded formulation of ER capsules, contains a mixture of 40% IR and 60% ER beads. Ritalin LA and its generic ER capsules are a combination of 50% IR and 50% DR beads. These products mimic BID dosing of IR. Cotempla delivers a mixture of 25% IR and 75% ER in an orally disintegrating extended-release formulation. Jornay PM is dosed in evening; if early-morning awakening occurs, dose earlier in evening.
- Concerta is based on the OROS osmotic delivery system (also used for Invega). 22% of the dose is immediate (with effects in one to two hours) and 78% is delayed. If you prescribe a generic, you may need to investigate carefully to ensure that the delivery system is an OROS pump system. To avoid insomnia, dosing should be completed by noon.

METHYLPHENIDATE TRANSDERMAL (Daytrana) Fact Sheet

BOTTOM LINE:
Daytrana is helpful for kids who, for whatever reason, cannot use any of the wide variety of oral stimulant preparations. Otherwise, we don't recommend it due to high cost, lag time for onset of effect, and the side effect of rash, which is pretty common and unpleasant.

PEDIATRIC FDA INDICATIONS:
ADHD (6–17 years).

ADULT FDA INDICATIONS:
ADHD.

DOSAGE FORMS:
Transdermal patch: 10 mg, 15 mg, 20 mg, 30 mg/9 hour.

PEDIATRIC DOSAGE GUIDANCE:
Start 10 mg/9 hour patch QAM (for initial therapy or for patients switching from other methylphenidate preparations, regardless of dose). Apply to hip two hours before an effect is needed and remove nine hours after application (drug effects may persist for five hours after removal). Increase dose at weekly intervals by using next-higher-dose system. May be removed in <9 hours if shorter duration is desired or if late-day side effects occur. Rotate application sites. Max 30 mg QD.

MONITORING: Weight, height, BP/P; ECG.

COST: $$$

SIDE EFFECTS:
- Most common: Headache, insomnia, irritability, decreased appetite, anorexia, nausea, tics, application site reaction (10%–40% incidence in children).
- Serious but rare: Allergic contact dermatitis/sensitization, characterized by intense local reactions (eg, edema, papules) that may spread beyond patch site; sensitization may subsequently manifest systemically with other routes of methylphenidate administration.

MECHANISM, PHARMACOKINETICS, AND DRUG INTERACTIONS:
- Stimulant that inhibits reuptake of dopamine and norepinephrine.
- Hepatic metabolism via carboxylesterase CES1A1, not CYP450 isoenzymes; t ½: 3–4 hours.
- Avoid use with MAOIs, antacids.

EVIDENCE AND CLINICAL PEARLS:
- FDA approved with several studies supporting its efficacy and safety, with a larger treatment effect size than non-stimulant medications, including in preschoolers (albeit no FDA indication for this age group).
- Apply patch to clean, dry area of the hip; don't apply to waistline or to areas under tight clothes, as it may rub off. Alternate sites daily (eg, opposite hip). Absorption not affected by perspiration. Remove after nine hours. If dislodged, replace with a new patch but remove within the nine-hour total wear time.
- Clinical effect usually seen in two hours and lasts approximately 12 hours.
- Exposure of application site to a heat source (eg, hair dryer, heating pad, electric blanket) may increase the amount of drug absorbed.
- For localized skin reactions (redness at site), use cortisone cream (1%–2%). For persistent, severe, or systemic reactions, discontinue patch.
- In June 2015, the FDA added a warning that Daytrana can cause chemical leukoderma, a permanent loss of skin color. These reactions are irreversible and not harmful but can be disfiguring to patients. Instruct patients to contact their physician if they notice skin color changes or lightening of skin areas; in such cases, an alternative medication should be considered.
- The manufacturer recommends to not cut the patch as it may release medication inconsistently or too quickly.

FUN FACT:
Since 2006, Shire Pharmaceuticals has issued at least 10 recalls of Daytrana patches because users have had difficulty removing the protective cover from the patch. Recall costs have reached into the millions.

MIXED AMPHETAMINE SALTS (Adderall, Adderall XR, Mydayis) Fact Sheet [G]

BOTTOM LINE:
Adderall is effective but is probably the most misused and diverted of all stimulants, and it tends to have more side effects, all of which is why we recommend starting most patients on methylphenidate instead.

PEDIATRIC FDA INDICATIONS:
ADHD (3–17 years for IR, 6–17 years for XR, 13–17 years for Mydayis); **narcolepsy** (6–17 years).

ADULT FDA INDICATIONS:
ADHD; narcolepsy.

OFF-LABEL USES:
Obesity; treatment-resistant depression.

DOSAGE FORMS:
- **Tablets (Adderall, [G]):** 5 mg, 7.5 mg, 10 mg, 12.5 mg, 15 mg, 20 mg, 30 mg.
- **ER capsules (Adderall XR, [G]):** 5 mg, 10 mg, 15 mg, 20 mg, 25 mg, 30 mg.
- **ER capsules (Mydayis):** 12.5 mg, 25 mg, 37.5 mg, 50 mg.

PEDIATRIC DOSAGE GUIDANCE:
- ADHD:
  - For IR and ER Adderall and its generic equivalent preparation. Initial dose should be 0.3 mg/kg/day, but shoot for a target dose of 1.0 mg/kg/day and maximum dose of 2 mg/kg/day.
  - IR (ages 3–5): Start 2.5 mg QAM, increase by 2.5 mg/day increments in weekly intervals, max 40 mg/day divided BID.
  - IR (ages 6–17): Start 5 mg QAM or BID, increase by 5 mg/day increments in weekly intervals, max 40 mg/day divided BID.
  - ER (ages 6–12): Start 5–10 mg QAM, increase by 5–10 mg/day increments weekly, 30 mg/day.
  - ER (ages 13–17): Start 10 mg QAM, increase by 10 mg/day increments weekly, max 40 mg/day QAM in adolescents.
  - Mydayis (adolescents 13–17 years): Start 12.5 mg QAM, increase in increments of 12.5 mg/day weekly, max 25 mg/day.
- Narcolepsy: Start 5 mg QAM (ages 6–11) or 10 mg QAM (ages 12–17), increase by 5 mg/day (ages 6–11) or 10 mg/day (ages 12–17) at weekly increments, max 60 mg/day.

MONITORING: Weight, height, BP/P; ECG.

COST: IR/ER: $; Mydayis: $$$$

SIDE EFFECTS:
- Most common: Insomnia, headache, decreased appetite, abdominal pain, weight loss, agitation.
- Serious but rare: See class warnings in chapter introduction.

MECHANISM, PHARMACOKINETICS, AND DRUG INTERACTIONS:
- Stimulant that inhibits reuptake of dopamine and norepinephrine.
- Metabolized primarily through CYP2D6; t ½: 9–14 hours. Duration of action: 6–8 hours (IR), 8–12 hours (XR).
- Avoid use with MAOIs, antacids. Caution with 2D6 inhibitors, which may increase stimulant effects.

EVIDENCE AND CLINICAL PEARLS:
- FDA approved with many studies and long history of clinical use supporting its efficacy and safety, with a larger treatment effect size than non-stimulant medications.
- Each dose contains a mixture of amphetamine salts, resulting in a 75:25 ratio of dextro and levo isomers of amphetamine.
- When converting from IR to ER, use the same total daily dose, given QAM.
- Adderall may provide more of a "kick" than methylphenidate preparations. Roughly twice as potent (per mg) as methylphenidate.
- Mydayis is formulated with pH-dependent drug-releasing beads, with immediate-release beads and delayed-release beads that release drug at pH 5.5 and pH 7.0. Duration of effect may be up to 16 hours.
- Dextroamphetamine and mixed amphetamine salts are the only stimulants approved for children <6 years (approved for children >3 years), with the exception of Mydayis, which causes very high rates of side effects (insomnia, reduced appetite) in children <13 years and should only be used in children ≥13 years.

FUN FACTS:
Was briefly pulled from the market in Canada in 2005 because of cardiac concerns, and now counterfeit Adderall is a common vehicle for overdose and death due to adulteration with fentanyl or methamphetamine.

VILOXAZINE XR (Qelbree) Fact Sheet

BOTTOM LINE:
Like the first norepinephrine reuptake inhibitor for ADHD, atomoxetine, viloxazine has no misuse potential and is less likely than stimulants to cause insomnia, anxiety, or tics. However, it is generally less effective than stimulants and takes longer to work. While viloxazine may work faster than atomoxetine, it's unclear if it has any advantage, and unlike atomoxetine, there's no option for a cheaper generic.

PEDIATRIC FDA INDICATIONS:
ADHD (6–17 years).

ADULT FDA INDICATIONS:
ADHD.

OFF-LABEL USES:
Treatment-resistant depression.

DOSAGE FORMS:
ER capsules: 100 mg, 150 mg, 200 mg.

PEDIATRIC DOSAGE GUIDANCE:
- Children >12: Start 200 mg QD, ↑ by 200 mg/day after one week to max 400 mg QD.
- Children 6–11: Start 100 mg QD, ↑ by 100 mg/day at weekly intervals to max 400 mg QD.

MONITORING: BP/P; baseline renal function.

COST: $$$$

SIDE EFFECTS:
- Most common: Somnolence, decreased appetite, fatigue, nausea, vomiting, insomnia, irritability.
- Serious but rare: Class warning for suicidal ideation in children and teens. Mania reported. May increase pulse and BP.

MECHANISM, PHARMACOKINETICS, AND DRUG INTERACTIONS:
- Selective norepinephrine reuptake inhibitor (NRI).
- Metabolized primarily via CYP2D6, UGT1A9, UGTB15; t ½: 7 hours.
- Avoid use with MAOIs. Strong 1A2 inhibitor; exercise caution with 1A2 substrates with narrow therapeutic index (eg, clozapine, duloxetine, ramelteon, tasimelteon, tizanidine, theophylline) as combination may increase side effects of substrate.

EVIDENCE AND CLINICAL PEARLS:
- ER capsules, so do not cut, crush, or chew; can open and sprinkle contents in applesauce.
- Adjust dose in severe renal impairment (eGFR <30 mL/min); max 200 mg/day.
- Data from one of four studies suggest viloxazine may work a bit faster than atomoxetine (week one vs week three), but this finding is not based on head-to-head data and it's hard to know whether it is clinically significant.
- Effective and FDA approved for ADHD; however, not likely to produce as robust of a treatment effect as stimulants.
- Of the two NRIs available for ADHD, atomoxetine is cheaper than viloxazine.

FUN FACT:
Viloxazine has been studied and rejected for various indications since the 1970s and originally received an FDA orphan drug designation for narcolepsy.

Antidepressants

In contrast to the data available for adults, the evidence for efficacy and safety of antidepressants in children is less robust. Nonetheless, some studies, specifically the TADS (Treatment for Adolescents With Depression Study) and TORDIA (Treatment of Resistant Depression in Adolescents), have shown that SSRIs can work for depression in adolescents, especially when combined with cognitive behavioral therapy. Recent meta-analyses continue to support this general guidance, particularly with fluoxetine. Data remain sparse regarding the safety and efficacy of newer antidepressants in the pediatric population.

Before considering an antidepressant trial, it is important to assess whether your patient either has bipolar disorder or is at higher risk for converting to bipolar disorder, as SSRIs often destabilize this population and require closer follow-up.

CHOOSING ANTIDEPRESSANTS

In general, when faced with a child or adolescent with depression who has not responded to psychotherapy, we recommend starting with fluoxetine, because it has the most evidence for efficacy and safety. Other first-line options include sertraline and escitalopram. Paroxetine has fallen out of favor due to concerns about suicidality as a possible side effect and significant withdrawal symptoms. Remember to start low and go slow, being mindful of the time needed for these medications to take effect.

If the first SSRI trial fails, rotate to a different SSRI. An SNRI trial (either venlafaxine or duloxetine) may be reasonable after two failed SSRI trials; however, SNRIs are not as effective as SSRIs in the pediatric population and are associated with more significant discontinuation symptoms.

Try bupropion for patients who have comorbid depression and ADHD, but remember that this medication lowers seizure threshold and has been associated with seizures in patients with bulimia. Mirtazapine and trazodone can be helpful for depressed and anxious patients with insomnia—but mirtazapine can cause substantial weight gain.

When antidepressants are not working well enough on their own, you can use augmenting agents, including second-generation antipsychotics, lithium, and thyroid supplementation. However, there is very little research evidence supporting this practice in the pediatric population.

We rarely use tricyclics in kids, because of possible cardiac toxicity and other side effects. Nonetheless, consider them for particularly severe and unresponsive cases, or for patients with comorbid OCD (esp. clomipramine), enuresis, insomnia, migraines, or poorly controlled headaches.

For treatment-resistant depression, small studies are promising but sparse for ketamine and transcranial magnetic stimulation (TMS), with significant financial considerations and a lack of large studies. Longer-term safety data are needed regarding the impact these options may have on developing brains.

DISCONTINUING ANTIDEPRESSANTS

When someone has responded well to an antidepressant, the general recommendation is that after six to 12 months of remission, we should begin a gradual tapering process over several weeks or a few months. Withdrawal is a common concern and may require a much slower tapering schedule. For patients with repeated depressive episodes, you will likely want to continue the medication. Patients do better if you take the tapering process slowly, if they have had effective psychotherapy that addresses life issues and/or gives them cognitive behavioral skills to manage their mood, and if they are not entering into a period of a major life change (eg, moving, school change, divorce). In cases where you need to abruptly discontinue medication due to hypomania, there is a far higher rate of withdrawal side effects.

SIDE EFFECTS AND CLASS WARNINGS

- Black box warning for suicidality: All antidepressant medications come with a black box warning based on a meta-analysis that demonstrated a two-fold increase in suicidal thinking or behaviors in patients under 25 years of age. No completed suicides were demonstrated, and the suicidal parameters encompassed a broad range of definitions, including parasuicidal thoughts and behaviors. We have studied this concern in detail and concluded that while antidepressants can be very helpful and reduce suicidality, there are some cases where these medications are associated with new or increased suicidality. Given this rare but significant risk, we have a duty to warn patients and families about this potential problem, and we need to monitor for it, particularly in the early stages of starting antidepressant medications.
- SSRIs:
  - The most common side effects of SSRIs include GI symptoms of nausea and diarrhea, which are typically transient and resolve for the majority of patients after several days. These can be minimized by starting with lower doses than usual.
  - Sleep disruptions and intense dreams can occur.
  - Children and adolescents are more sensitive to activation and restlessness than adults.
  - Carbohydrate craving is fairly common in patients taking SSRIs.

- Citalopram and (to a lesser extent) escitalopram increase QT in a dose-dependent manner.
- Increased bleeding due to platelet inhibition can occur with SSRIs and other serotonergic antidepressants.
- Gradual tapers are required (with the exception of fluoxetine, given its long half-life) to avoid discontinuation symptoms, which most often occur with paroxetine. While not dangerous, discontinuation syndrome can be extremely uncomfortable and may include nausea, diarrhea, "brain zaps," headache, and irritability, to name a few symptoms.
- SNRIs:
  - Given their potential to increase blood pressure, closer blood pressure monitoring is required.
  - Gradual tapers are also required, considering SNRIs' significant withdrawal symptoms.
- Other side effect considerations:
  - Serotonin syndrome can occur, particularly when using multiple serotonergic agents including supplements such as St. John's wort and S-adenosyl-L-methionine (SAMe), over-the-counter cough preparations containing dextromethorphan, or methylenedioxymethamphetamine (also known as MDMA or ecstasy); if it occurs, it will require discontinuation of offending medications or supplements. Symptoms often present within a day of starting medication and can include sweating, GI symptoms, hyperthermia, tachycardia, increased blood pressure, confusion, and tremors. These symptoms can be life threatening and will require immediate assessment and supportive care.
  - Risks of hypomania and mania need to be considered.
  - Sexual side effects are common, including delayed orgasm/ejaculation and decreased sexual drive, which may be of concern to some adolescents—bupropion and mirtazapine are less likely to cause these problems.

Depressive Disorders Treatment Algorithm for Children and Adolescents

*Denotes off label

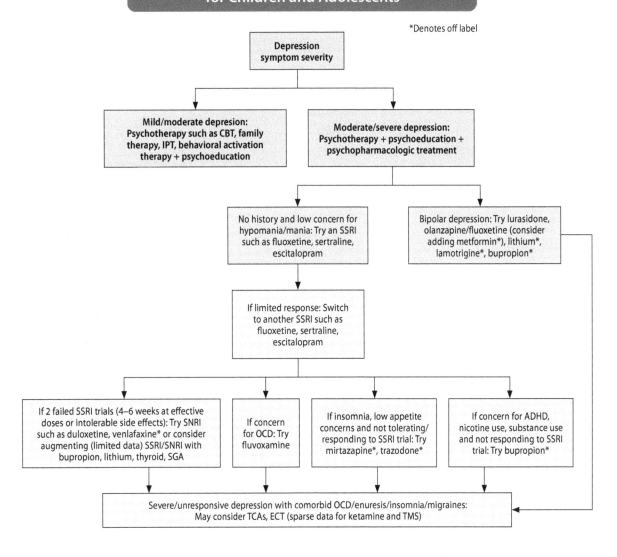

Depression symptom severity

Mild/moderate depresion: Psychotherapy such as CBT, family therapy, IPT, behavioral activation therapy + psychoeducation

Moderate/severe depression: Psychotherapy + psychoeducation + psychopharmacologic treatment

No history and low concern for hypomania/mania: Try an SSRI such as fluoxetine, sertraline, escitalopram

Bipolar depression: Try lurasidone, olanzapine/fluoxetine (consider adding metformin*), lithium*, lamotrigine*, bupropion*

If limited response: Switch to another SSRI such as fluoxetine, sertraline, escitalopram

If 2 failed SSRI trials (4–6 weeks at effective doses or intolerable side effects): Try SNRI such as duloxetine, venlafaxine* or consider augmenting (limited data) SSRI/SNRI with bupropion, lithium, thyroid, SGA

If concern for OCD: Try fluvoxamine

If insomnia, low appetite concerns and not tolerating/responding to SSRI trial: Try mirtazapine*, trazodone*

If concern for ADHD, nicotine use, substance use and not responding to SSRI trial: Try bupropion*

Severe/unresponsive depression with comorbid OCD/enuresis/insomnia/migraines: May consider TCAs, ECT (sparse data for ketamine and TMS)

- Use non-pharmacologic approaches first when possible to help reduce use of medication
- See text and tables for specific age-related guidance
- If using antidepressants, discuss potential side effects including rare but possible increase in behavioral activation or suicidal thinking
- If using antipsychotics, check weight and labs (lipids, HbA1c, others as indicated) at baseline, 12 weeks, and yearly or sooner, AIMS at baseline and every 6 months or sooner, and consider ECG at baseline and yearly or sooner
- If stable for 6–12 months, consider gradual taper and discontinuation of medications

Key

CBT – Cognitive behavioral therapy
IPT – Interpersonal psychotherapy
SGA – Second-generation antipsychotic
TCA – Tricyclic antidepressants
TMS – Transcranial magnetic stimulation therapy

Antidepressants

CARLAT PUBLISHING © 2023

TABLE 3: Antidepressants

Generic Name (Brand Name) Year FDA Approved [G] denotes generic availability	Relevant FDA Indication(s) (Pediatric indications in bold)	Available Strengths (mg)	Usual Dosage Range (starting–max) (mg) *Pediatric unless specified*
Selective Serotonin Reuptake Inhibitors (SSRIs)			
Citalopram [G] (Celexa) 1998	MDD	10, 20, 40, 10/5 mL	10–40
Escitalopram [G] (Lexapro) 2002	**MDD (12+ yrs)**, GAD	5, 10, 20, 5/5 mL	5–20
Fluoxetine [G] (Prozac) 1987	**MDD (8+ yrs), OCD (7+ yrs)**, panic disorder, bulimia, PMDD (as Sarafem)	10, 20, 40, 60, 20/5 mL	10–60
Fluoxetine DR [G] (Prozac Weekly) 2001	MDD maintenance	90 DR	90 Q week (adults)
Fluvoxamine [G] Luvox brand discontinued; generic only 1994	**OCD (8+ yrs)**	25, 50, 100	50–300
Fluvoxamine ER [G] (Luvox CR) 2008	OCD	100, 150 ER	100–300
Paroxetine [G] (Paxil) 1992 (Pexeva) 2003 (Brisdelle) 2013	MDD, OCD, panic disorder, social anxiety, GAD, PTSD, PMDD, menopausal hot flashes (as Brisdelle)	7.5 (Brisdelle), 10, 20, 30, 40, 10/5 mL	10–60
Paroxetine CR [G] (Paxil CR) 1999	MDD, panic disorder, social anxiety, PMDD	12.5, 25, 37.5 ER	12.5–62.5
Sertraline [G] (Zoloft) 1991	MDD, **OCD (6+ yrs)**, panic disorder, PTSD, PMDD, social anxiety	25, 50, 100, 150, 200, 20/mL	12.5–200
Serotonin Norepinephrine Reuptake Inhibitors (SNRIs)			
Desvenlafaxine [G] (Pristiq) 2008	MDD	25, 50, 100 ER	50–100 (adults)
Duloxetine [G] (Cymbalta) 2004 (Drizalma Sprinkle) 2019	MDD, **GAD (7+ yrs)** (also diabetic peripheral neuropathy, fibromyalgia, chronic musculoskeletal pain)	20, 30, 40, 60 DR	30–120
Venlafaxine [G] 1993 Effexor brand discontinued; generic only	MDD	25, 37.5, 50, 75, 100	37.5–75
Venlafaxine ER [G] (Effexor XR) 1997	MDD, GAD, social anxiety disorder, panic disorder	37.5, 75, 150, 225 ER	37.5–225
Tricyclic Antidepressants (TCAs)			
Amitriptyline [G] Elavil brand discontinued; generic only 1961	MDD	10, 25, 50, 75, 100, 150	25–200
Clomipramine [G] (Anafranil) 1989	**OCD (10+ yrs)**	25, 50, 75	25–200
Desipramine [G] (Norpramin) 1964	MDD	10, 25, 50, 75, 100, 150	25–150

Generic Name (Brand Name) Year FDA Approved *[G] denotes generic availability*	Relevant FDA Indication(s) (Pediatric indications in bold)	Available Strengths (mg)	Usual Dosage Range (starting–max) (mg) *Pediatric unless specified*
Imipramine [G] Tofranil brand discontinued; generic only 1984	MDD	10, 25, 50, 75, 100, 125, 150	10–100
Nortriptyline [G] (Pamelor) 1977	MDD	10, 25, 50, 75, 10/5 mL	10–150
Monoamine Oxidase Inhibitor (MAOI)			
Selegiline transdermal (EMSAM) 2006	MDD	6, 9, 12/24-hr patch	6–12/24 hrs (adults)
Dopamine Norepinephrine Reuptake Inhibitors			
Bupropion [G] (Wellbutrin) 1985	MDD	75, 100	100–450
Bupropion SR [G] (Wellbutrin SR) 1996	MDD, smoking cessation	100, 150, 200	100–400
Bupropion XL [G] (Wellbutrin XL, Forfivo XL) 2003	MDD, seasonal affective disorder	150, 300 (Wellbutrin XL), 450 (Forfivo XL)	150–450
Noradrenergic and Specific Serotonergic Antidepressants (NaSSAs)			
Mirtazapine [G] (Remeron) 1996	MDD	7.5, 15, 30, 45	7.5–45
Mirtazapine ODT [G] (Remeron SolTab) 2001	MDD	15, 30, 45	7.5–45
Serotonin Reuptake Inhibitor and 5-HT2A and 5-HT2C Antagonist			
Trazodone [G] Desyrel brand discontinued; generic only 1981	MDD	50, 100, 150, 300	25–400

Antidepressants

BUPROPION (Wellbutrin, others) Fact Sheet [G]

BOTTOM LINE:
Not a first-line antidepressant in kids, but may be useful for kids whose depression is associated with fatigue and poor concentration. Absence of sexual side effects and weight gain make this an appealing option for some. Although not effective for anxiety disorders, it is effective for the anxiety that often accompanies depression. The seizure risk is not a concern for most patients when dosed appropriately.

PEDIATRIC FDA INDICATIONS:
None.

ADULT FDA INDICATIONS:
Major depression; seasonal affective disorder; smoking cessation (as Zyban).

OFF-LABEL USES:
ADHD; sexual dysfunction; bipolar depression.

DOSAGE FORMS:
* **Tablets (G):** 75 mg, 100 mg.
* **SR tablets (G):** 100 mg, 150 mg, 200 mg.
* **ER tablets (G):** 150 mg, 300 mg; **Forfivo XL:** 450 mg.
* **ER tablets, hydrobromide salt formulation (Aplenzin):** 174 mg, 348 mg, 522 mg (equivalent to 150 mg, 300 mg, 450 mg, respectively).

PEDIATRIC DOSAGE GUIDANCE:
* Depression (target dose 300 mg/day):
  – IR: Start 37.5 mg or 75 mg BID, ↑ to TID after >3 days; max dose 450 mg/day, 150 mg/dose; separate doses by at least six hours to minimize seizure risk.
  – SR: Start 100 mg QAM, ↑ to 100 mg BID as early as fourth day; max dose 400 mg/day, 200 mg/dose; separate doses by at least eight hours to minimize seizure risk.
  – ER: Start 150 mg QAM, ↑ to 300 mg QAM as early as fourth day; max dose 450 mg QAM.
* Smoking cessation: Start 100 mg SR QAM, titrate as needed.

MONITORING: No routine monitoring recommended unless clinical picture warrants.

COST: IR/SR/ER: $; Forfivo: $$$; Aplenzin: $$$$$

SIDE EFFECTS:
* Most common: Agitation, irritability, insomnia, headache, nausea, vomiting, tremor, tachycardia, dry mouth, weight loss.
* Serious but rare: Seizures; risk higher with rapid and large dose increases and in patients at risk for seizures. Risk of seizure depends on dose and formulation: IR: 0.4% at 300–450 mg/day vs 4% at 450–600 mg/day. SR/ER: 0.1% at 100–300 mg/day vs 0.4% at 400 mg/day. Do not chew, divide, or crush SR or ER tablets as risk of seizures may be increased.

MECHANISM, PHARMACOKINETICS, AND DRUG INTERACTIONS:
* Dopamine and norepinephrine receptor uptake inhibitor.
* Metabolized primarily through CYP2B6; inhibits CYP2D6; t ½: 21 hours.
* Avoid use with MAOIs.

EVIDENCE AND CLINICAL PEARLS:
* Although used clinically by some child psychiatrists, support for bupropion's efficacy in depression is based on one study in kids with comorbid ADHD and one open trial in adolescents with depression.
* For treatment of ADHD, a few head-to-head studies found bupropion to be equally effective as methylphenidate, but a large placebo-controlled trial found smaller effect sizes for bupropion.
* May be a particularly good option for kids with comorbid illness, such as ADHD or tobacco use disorder.
* There are only a few studies of bupropion for smoking cessation in adolescents. One study found bupropion provided no benefit when added to nicotine patches vs using patch alone. But another study showed improved quit rates (though lower than in adults) when combined with counseling vs counseling alone.
* Forfivo XL offers ease of use (one pill a day) for patients taking 450 mg/day, but it is more expensive. Aplenzin brand could also be a one-pill-a-day solution (522 mg is equivalent to 450 mg Wellbutrin) but otherwise doesn't offer any real advantage as a different salt (hydrobromide).
* Give ER dose as early in the morning as possible to minimize insomnia.
* Bupropion can cause false-positive urine test results for amphetamines.

NOT-SO-FUN FACT:
There have been case reports of teenagers, prisoners, and others snorting crushed tablets (believing the substance to be a stimulant), with subsequent seizures.

CITALOPRAM (Celexa) Fact Sheet [G]

BOTTOM LINE:
Citalopram does not have any pediatric indications, and its efficacy data are limited and modest; however, it is a reasonable second-line off-label SSRI option.

PEDIATRIC FDA INDICATIONS:
None.

ADULT FDA INDICATIONS:
Major depression.

OFF-LABEL USES:
OCD; major depression; PTSD; social anxiety; GAD; panic disorder; PMDD.

DOSAGE FORMS:
- **Tablets (G):** 10 mg, 20 mg (scored), 40 mg (scored).
- **Oral solution (G):** 10 mg/5 mL.

PEDIATRIC DOSAGE GUIDANCE:
- Minimal dosing guidance in children and adolescents.
- Ages 7–11: Start 10 mg QD, increase by 5 mg/day increments every one to two weeks; max 40 mg/day.
- Ages 12–17: Start 10 mg or 20 mg QD, increase by 10 mg/day increments every one to two weeks; max 40 mg/day.
- Most patients take it in the morning, but bedtime dosing is OK if there is no insomnia.

MONITORING: ECG in patients on >40 mg/day.

COST: $

SIDE EFFECTS:
- Most common: Nausea, insomnia, anxiety, sexual side effects, apathy, headache.
- Serious but rare: Hyponatremia, mainly in the elderly; gastrointestinal bleeding, especially when combined with NSAIDs such as ibuprofen.

MECHANISM, PHARMACOKINETICS, AND DRUG INTERACTIONS:
- Selective serotonin reuptake inhibitor.
- Metabolized primarily through CYP2C19 and 3A4; t ½: 35 hours.
- Avoid use with MAOIs (allow a two-week washout period); avoid other serotonergic agents (serotonin syndrome).
- Use caution in patients taking CYP2C19 inhibitors (eg, cimetidine, omeprazole), which will increase citalopram levels and potential for QT prolongation.

EVIDENCE AND CLINICAL PEARLS:
- A 12-week randomized double-blind European study of 244 adolescents with depression found no significant difference in improvement between citalopram and placebo. When patients receiving psychotherapy were excluded from analysis, there were significantly higher response and remission rates with citalopram than placebo.
- Another eight-week randomized double-blind trial in 174 children and adolescents with depression found citalopram response rates low (36%), but significantly higher than placebo (24%).
- Citalopram's maximum daily dose was reduced to 40 mg/day by the FDA in August 2011 due to data suggesting increased QTc interval prolongation at doses >40 mg/day. Mean QTc interval prolongation at 60 mg/day was 18.5 msec (vs ziprasidone, which has been shown to increase this interval by 20.6 msec).
- Use lower doses and max 20 mg/day in patients deemed to be poor CYP2C19 metabolizers.

FUN FACT:
A parody prescription drug commercial by the website *Funny or Die* is based on a combination of real-life clozapine and citalopram. The tagline is "DredLexa: the first depressant for rappers—sad music is better music."

Antidepressants

DESVENLAFAXINE (Pristiq) Fact Sheet [G]

BOTTOM LINE:
There are no clear advantages to using desvenlafaxine over other agents, particularly venlafaxine XR. Given minimal data in kids, we'd stick with venlafaxine if deciding to go with an SNRI.

PEDIATRIC FDA INDICATIONS:
None.

ADULT FDA INDICATIONS:
Major depression.

OFF-LABEL USES:
Fibromyalgia; GAD; social anxiety disorder; panic disorder; PTSD; PMDD.

DOSAGE FORMS:
ER tablets (G): 25 mg, 50 mg, 100 mg.

PEDIATRIC DOSAGE GUIDANCE:
Start 25 mg QD. Increase to 50 mg QD based on response and tolerability. May increase to 100 mg QD in adolescents, but higher doses are generally not more effective and may be less well tolerated.

MONITORING: Periodic BP.

COST: $

SIDE EFFECTS:
- Most common: Nausea, dizziness, insomnia, excessive sweating, constipation, dry mouth, somnolence, decreased appetite, anxiety, sexual side effects.
- Serious but rare: Dose-related increases in systolic and diastolic blood pressure (as likely with desvenlafaxine as venlafaxine). Monitor BP regularly, and if increases are sustained, consider reducing dose or discontinuing.

MECHANISM, PHARMACOKINETICS, AND DRUG INTERACTIONS:
- Serotonin and norepinephrine reuptake inhibitor.
- Active metabolite of venlafaxine, metabolized primarily through conjugation and oxidation via CYP3A4 (minor). Minimally inhibits CYP2D6; t ½: 11 hours.
- Avoid use with MAOIs and other serotonergic medications. Not likely to cause other clinically significant interactions.

EVIDENCE AND CLINICAL PEARLS:
- Minimal data in kids with depression (one open-label study of 20 children and 20 adolescents that looked at safety and tolerability only, not efficacy).
- A recent randomized double-blind placebo-controlled study of over 300 kids with depression showed desvenlafaxine was no better than placebo.
- Desvenlafaxine has not been shown to be any more effective than venlafaxine. Unlike venlafaxine, increasing the dose of desvenlafaxine beyond the recommended 50 mg/day likely does not improve response, but does increase side effects.
- Claims of fewer drug interactions with desvenlafaxine are likely unimportant for the majority of patients as the risk of clinically significant interactions with venlafaxine is already quite low.
- Desvenlafaxine is available in two forms: a succinate salt (Pristiq) and a base (previously branded as Khedezla). Aside from small differences in half-life, there is no difference between these products—all efficacy studies were based on the original Pristiq studies.

FUN FACT:
Desvenlafaxine's manufacturer withdrew its application for approval in the European Union, where regulatory bodies said that desvenlafaxine was likely less effective than venlafaxine with no advantages in terms of safety and tolerability.

DULOXETINE (Cymbalta, Drizalma Sprinkle) Fact Sheet [G]

BOTTOM LINE:
Mixed data and possibly more side effects versus SSRIs (BP, P) relegate this to second-line status for treating kids with depression. But consider in kids with GAD or in those with depression who have failed alternatives or who have comorbid pain disorders.

PEDIATRIC FDA INDICATIONS:
GAD (7–17 years).

ADULT FDA INDICATIONS:
Major depression; GAD; diabetic peripheral neuropathic pain; fibromyalgia; chronic musculoskeletal pain (including osteoarthritis and chronic low back pain).

OFF-LABEL USES:
Other neuropathic or chronic pain disorders; other anxiety disorders; stress urinary incontinence.

DOSAGE FORMS:
Delayed-release capsules (Cymbalta, Drizalma Sprinkle, [G]): 20 mg, 30 mg, 40 mg, 60 mg.

PEDIATRIC DOSAGE GUIDANCE:
- GAD: Start 30 mg QD, increase by 30 mg/day after two weeks; max dose 60 mg QD.
- Depression: Minimal data in kids; follow GAD dosing recommendations.
- Dose timing depends on patient preference since it causes drowsiness in some but insomnia in others. Let patients/families experiment until they get it right.

MONITORING: Periodic BP.

COST: $; Drizalma Sprinkle: $$$

SIDE EFFECTS:
- Most common: Nausea, dry mouth, constipation, diarrhea, decreased appetite, vomiting, fatigue, insomnia, dizziness, agitation, sweating, headache, urinary hesitation, sexual side effects.
- Serious but rare: Rare cases of hepatic failure (including fatalities) have been reported (too rare to require routine LFTs in all patients). Hepatitis with abdominal pain, hepatomegaly, elevated transaminases >20 times normal with and without jaundice observed. May cause orthostatic hypotension or syncope, especially in first week of therapy and after dose increases. Urinary retention reported; hospitalization and/or catheterization were necessary in some cases.

MECHANISM, PHARMACOKINETICS, AND DRUG INTERACTIONS:
- Serotonin and norepinephrine reuptake inhibitor.
- Metabolized primarily through CYP1A2 and 2D6; inhibitor of CYP2D6; t ½: 12 hours.
- Avoid use with MAOIs and other serotonergic medications. Caution with drugs metabolized by CYP2D6 (eg, paroxetine, fluoxetine, aripiprazole, iloperidone, risperidone, atomoxetine, beta-blockers) as their levels may be increased. Potent inhibitors of CYP2D6 (eg, paroxetine, fluoxetine, quinidine) and CYP1A2 (eg, fluvoxamine, ciprofloxacin) may increase duloxetine levels.

EVIDENCE AND CLINICAL PEARLS:
- Two placebo-controlled studies of 8,000 kids with depression didn't show efficacy. Two safety studies showed expected side effects in kids of increased BP and pulse, nausea, and headache.
- A more recent meta-analysis in depressed kids was more promising; however, the data for duloxetine were considered to be of low quality.
- Since capsules are delayed release, they should be swallowed whole; do not chew or crush. Although the manufacturer does not recommend opening the capsules, their contents may be sprinkled on applesauce or in apple juice and swallowed immediately.
- Avoid in patients with a history of heavy alcohol use or chronic hepatic disease because of the possibility that duloxetine and alcohol may interact, causing hepatic injury, or the possibility that duloxetine may aggravate preexisting hepatic disease.
- Drizalma Sprinkle is a new formulation for use in patients with swallowing difficulty, either by sprinkling over applesauce or administering via nasogastric tube.

FUN FACT:
Duloxetine is approved in Europe for stress urinary incontinence, but the FDA refused this indication in the US because of concerns regarding liver toxicity and potential suicidal ideation.

ESCITALOPRAM (Lexapro) Fact Sheet [G]

BOTTOM LINE:
Although only one of three randomized controlled trials led to FDA approval in adolescents, due to the general lack of effective options you may consider escitalopram a first-line agent, particularly in adolescents with depression and anxiety disorders. Efficacy of escitalopram in OCD and other anxiety disorders has not been established; for those, stick to fluoxetine or sertraline.

PEDIATRIC FDA INDICATIONS:
Major depression (12+ years).

ADULT FDA INDICATIONS:
Major depression; GAD.

OFF-LABEL USES:
OCD; PTSD; social anxiety; panic disorder; PMDD; autism.

DOSAGE FORMS:
* **Tablets (G):** 5 mg, 10 mg (scored), 20 mg (scored).
* **Oral solution (G):** 5 mg/5 mL.

PEDIATRIC DOSAGE GUIDANCE:
* Ages 6–9: Start 2.5 mg QD, increase by 5 mg/day increments weekly; max 20 mg/day.
* Ages 10–17: Start 5 mg QD, increase by 5–10 mg/day increments weekly; max 20 mg/day.
* Dose timing is generally in the morning due to good tolerability, but it could be taken at any time of day.

MONITORING: ECG in patients on >20 mg/day.

COST: $

SIDE EFFECTS:
* Most common: Nausea, insomnia, anxiety, sedation, sexual side effects, weight gain, apathy, headache.
* Serious but rare: Hyponatremia, mainly in the elderly; gastrointestinal bleeding, especially when combined with NSAIDs such as ibuprofen.

MECHANISM, PHARMACOKINETICS, AND DRUG INTERACTIONS:
* Selective serotonin reuptake inhibitor.
* Metabolized primarily through CYP2C19 and 3A4; t ½: 27–32 hours.
* Avoid use with MAOIs (allow a two-week washout period); avoid other serotonergic agents (serotonin syndrome).

EVIDENCE AND CLINICAL PEARLS:
* An eight-week randomized clinical trial of 268 children (ages 6–17) with depression failed to find a significant difference between escitalopram and placebo on primary outcome measures. When data analysis included only adolescent subjects, there was a significant difference in favor of escitalopram.
* Another eight-week randomized clinical trial of 312 adolescents showed only a small to medium effect size (0.27) on primary outcome measures of depression.
* FDA approval for adolescents with depression is based on one randomized double-blind placebo-controlled study in pediatric depression showing significantly greater efficacy compared to placebo.
* Escitalopram (which is purified from the racemic mixture, citalopram) is considered the "purest" SSRI and has few, if any, drug-drug interactions.

FUN FACT:
In his rap song "FML," Kanye West refers to "nothing crazier" than when "he off his Lexapro."

FLUOXETINE (Prozac, Prozac Weekly) Fact Sheet [G]

BOTTOM LINE:
Consider fluoxetine a first-line agent for kids with depression and anxiety disorders.

PEDIATRIC FDA INDICATIONS:
Major depression (8+ years); **OCD** (7+ years).

ADULT FDA INDICATIONS:
Major depression; OCD; panic disorder; bulimia; PMDD (as Sarafem).

OFF-LABEL USES:
PTSD; social anxiety; cataplexy.

DOSAGE FORMS:
- **Capsules (G):** 10 mg, 20 mg, 40 mg.
- **Tablets (G):** 10 mg, 20 mg, 60 mg.
- **Delayed-release capsules (Prozac Weekly, [G]):** 90 mg.
- **Oral solution (G):** 20 mg/5 mL.

PEDIATRIC DOSAGE GUIDANCE:
- Ages 6–7: Start 5 mg QD, increase by 5 mg/day increments weekly; max 30 mg/day.
- Ages 8–17: Start 10 mg QD, increase by 10 mg/day increments weekly; max 60 mg/day.
- Many children and adolescents will show good treatment response at 10 mg/day.
- Most will respond best to morning dosing given its activating effects.

MONITORING: No routine monitoring recommended unless clinical picture warrants.

COST: $; DR capsule: $$

SIDE EFFECTS:
- Most common: Nausea, insomnia, anxiety, sexual side effects, apathy, headache.
- Serious but rare: Hyponatremia, mainly in the elderly; gastrointestinal bleeding, especially when combined with NSAIDs such as ibuprofen.

MECHANISM, PHARMACOKINETICS, AND DRUG INTERACTIONS:
- Selective serotonin reuptake inhibitor.
- Metabolized primarily through CYP2D6; potent CYP2C9/19 and 2D6 inhibitor; moderate CYP3A4 inhibitor; t ½: 4–6 days (9 days for norfluoxetine metabolite).
- Avoid use with MAOIs (allow a five-week washout period if switching to MAOI); avoid other serotonergic agents (serotonin syndrome). Caution with substrates of 2C9/19 and 2D6.

EVIDENCE AND CLINICAL PEARLS:
- Most studied SSRI in kids and the only antidepressant approved for treating depression in younger children.
- Two large randomized double-blind placebo-controlled trials that showed significantly greater efficacy for depression compared to placebo led to FDA indication in kids 8 and older.
- Fluoxetine is favored in patients who could use some activation; it is most likely to cause insomnia, anxiety, and decreased appetite.
- Generally, higher doses of SSRIs are required for treating OCD.

FUN FACT:
According to *National Geographic*, shrimp exposed to traces of fluoxetine swim in brighter areas, making them more vulnerable to predators. This fact is not so fun for the shrimp.

FLUVOXAMINE (Luvox, Luvox CR) Fact Sheet [G]

BOTTOM LINE:
Fluvoxamine was the first SSRI approved for OCD in children as young as 8. We favor fluoxetine and sertraline for ease of dosing, better tolerability, generally lower drug interaction potential, and lower likelihood for discontinuation syndrome.

PEDIATRIC FDA INDICATIONS:
OCD (8+ years).

ADULT FDA INDICATIONS:
OCD.

OFF-LABEL USES:
Major depression; panic disorder; GAD; PTSD.

DOSAGE FORMS:
- **Tablets (G):** 25 mg, 50 mg (scored), 100 mg (scored).
- **ER capsules (G):** 100 mg, 150 mg.

PEDIATRIC DOSAGE GUIDANCE:
- IR: Start 25 mg QHS, increase by 25 mg/day increments weekly; max 200 mg/day in ages 8–11 and 300 mg/day in ages >11. Doses >50 mg/day should be divided BID.
- ER (off-label for pediatric): Start 100 mg QHS, increase by 50 mg/day increments weekly; max (adults) 300 mg/day.

MONITORING: No routine monitoring recommended unless clinical picture warrants.

COST: $; ER: $$

SIDE EFFECTS:
- Most common: Nausea, sedation, sexual side effects, weight gain, apathy, headache.
- Serious but rare: Hyponatremia, mainly in the elderly; gastrointestinal bleeding, especially when combined with NSAIDs such as ibuprofen.

MECHANISM, PHARMACOKINETICS, AND DRUG INTERACTIONS:
- Selective serotonin reuptake inhibitor.
- Metabolized primarily through CYP1A2 and 2D6; potent inhibitor of CYP1A2 and 2C19; moderate inhibitor of 2C9 and 3A4; t ½: 16 hours.
- Avoid use with MAOIs (allow a two-week washout period); avoid other serotonergic agents (serotonin syndrome). Caution with substrates of CYP1A2 and 2C19.

EVIDENCE AND CLINICAL PEARLS:
- An eight-week placebo-controlled trial of 128 children (6–17 years) with social phobia, separation anxiety disorder, or GAD found significantly greater improvement on anxiety measures with fluvoxamine compared to placebo.
- A 10-week placebo-controlled trial of 120 children and adolescents (8–17 years) with OCD showed significantly higher reduction in Children's Yale-Brown Obsessive Compulsive Scale scores with fluvoxamine compared to placebo.
- There are no high-quality studies of fluvoxamine in children with depression.
- Fluvoxamine is used less often due to twice-daily dosing, risk for drug interactions, and fewer data for uses other than OCD, even though it's likely just as effective as other SSRIs.
- Discontinuation symptoms tend to be worse with fluvoxamine compared to other SSRIs.
- Generally, higher doses of SSRIs are required for treating OCD.

FUN FACT:
Families of victims of the Columbine shooting sued Luvox's manufacturer after it was revealed one of the shooters was taking this antidepressant.

MIRTAZAPINE (Remeron) Fact Sheet [G]

BOTTOM LINE:
Second- or third-line agent due to lack of data. Weight gain and sedation may limit its use in many kids. It may be useful in depressed patients with anxiety or insomnia, those who have had sexual side effects with other antidepressants, and those who may benefit from appetite stimulation.

PEDIATRIC FDA INDICATIONS:
None.

ADULT FDA INDICATIONS:
Major depression.

OFF-LABEL USES:
Panic disorder; PTSD; GAD; insomnia; nausea; appetite stimulant; methamphetamine use disorder.

DOSAGE FORMS:
- **Tablets (G):** 7.5 mg, 15 mg, 30 mg, 45 mg.
- **Orally disintegrating tablets (G):** 15 mg, 30 mg, 45 mg.

PEDIATRIC DOSAGE GUIDANCE:
- Very limited dosing guidance in children and adolescents.
- Start 7.5 mg or 15 mg QHS, ↑ by 15 mg/day every one to two weeks. Max 45 mg/day.

MONITORING: Weight.

COST: $

SIDE EFFECTS:
- Most common: Somnolence, increased appetite, weight gain, perhaps offset by stimulating effects of higher dosages.
- Serious but rare: Agranulocytosis or severe neutropenia (with or without infection) reported very rarely.

MECHANISM, PHARMACOKINETICS, AND DRUG INTERACTIONS:
- Noradrenergic (via central presynaptic alpha-2 adrenergic receptor antagonist activity) and specific serotonergic (via postsynaptic 5HT2 and 5HT3 antagonist effects) antidepressant.
- Metabolized primarily through CYP1A2, 2D6, and 3A4; t ½: 20–40 hours.
- Avoid use with MAOIs. Caution with inducers of 1A2 or 3A4 (eg, carbamazepine), which could reduce efficacy of mirtazapine.

EVIDENCE AND CLINICAL PEARLS:
- Two unpublished eight-week randomized trials of mirtazapine 15–45 mg/day in outpatient children and adolescents with depression found no significant reduction in depressive symptoms compared to placebo.
- One open-label 85-day study of mirtazapine 30–45 mg/day in 24 adolescents with depression showed marked efficacy on depression, anxiety, and sleep as well as good tolerability (sedation, weight gain, and increased appetite were most common side effects).
- Twenty-six subjects with pervasive developmental disorder (PDD) ages 4–24 years were treated with mirtazapine 7.5–45 mg/day in an open-label trial, showing only modest benefit for symptoms associated with autism and other PDD.
- If patients experience too much sedation at initial lower dose, increase dose; mirtazapine has increased noradrenergic effect relative to antihistaminergic effect at higher doses.
- Two small studies in adult men with methamphetamine use disorder have shown promising effects with reducing use.

FUN FACT:
Esmirtazapine, the (S)-enantiomer, was under development for the treatment of insomnia and hot flashes associated with menopause, but the company pulled the plug in 2010.

Antidepressants

PAROXETINE (Paxil, Paxil CR, Pexeva) Fact Sheet [G]

BOTTOM LINE:
Lack of efficacy, side effects, and discontinuation symptoms make paroxetine less appealing for children with depression.

PEDIATRIC FDA INDICATIONS:
None.

ADULT FDA INDICATIONS:
Major depression; OCD; panic disorder; social anxiety; GAD; PTSD; PMDD; menopausal hot flashes (as Brisdelle).

OFF-LABEL USES:
Premature ejaculation.

DOSAGE FORMS:
- **Tablets (Paxil, Pexeva, [G]):** 10 mg, 20 mg, 30 mg, 40 mg.
- **Oral suspension [G]:** 10 mg/5 mL.
- **ER tablets (Paxil CR, [G]):** 12.5 mg, 25 mg, 37.5 mg.
- **Capsules (Brisdelle, [G]):** 7.5 mg.

PEDIATRIC DOSAGE GUIDANCE:
- Minimal dosing guidance in children and adolescents.
- Start tablets/oral suspension 10 mg QD, increase by 10 mg/day increments every one to two weeks; max 60 mg/day.
- Start CR 12.5 mg QD, increase by 12.5 mg/day increments every one to two weeks; max 62.5 mg/day.
- Usually best given at bedtime due to sedation.

MONITORING: No routine monitoring recommended unless clinical picture warrants.

COST: $; liquid: $$$

SIDE EFFECTS:
- Most common: Nausea, sedation, anxiety, constipation, sexual side effects, weight gain, apathy, headache.
- Serious but rare: Hyponatremia, mainly in the elderly; gastrointestinal bleeding, especially when combined with NSAIDs such as ibuprofen.

MECHANISM, PHARMACOKINETICS, AND DRUG INTERACTIONS:
- Selective serotonin reuptake inhibitor.
- Metabolized primarily through CYP2D6; potent inhibitor of CYP2D6; t ½: 21 hours.
- Avoid use with MAOIs (allow a two-week washout period); avoid other serotonergic agents (serotonin syndrome). Caution with substrates of 2D6.

EVIDENCE AND CLINICAL PEARLS:
- Study 329, a 2001 study comparing paroxetine to imipramine in kids with depression, became controversial when it was found not only that the study had been ghostwritten by a PR firm hired by the drug manufacturer, but also that it made inappropriate claims about efficacy and downplayed safety concerns. A re-analysis published in 2015 found that neither paroxetine nor imipramine were better than placebo for depression and that paroxetine patients experienced more suicidal ideation and behavior while imipramine patients experienced more cardiovascular problems.
- A meta-analysis of four paroxetine trials in kids with depression found similar response and remission rates with placebo.
- Of the SSRIs, paroxetine is least favored due to its side effect profile (greatest sexual side effects, weight gain, sedation, constipation) and drug interaction profile.
- Discontinuation symptoms tend to be worse with paroxetine compared to other SSRIs.

FUN FACT:
New Scientist wrote in 2015: "You may never have heard of it, but Study 329 changed medicine." (See "Evidence and Clinical Pearls" section above.)

SELEGILINE TRANSDERMAL (EMSAM) Fact Sheet

BOTTOM LINE:
Minimal efficacy data in pediatric patients, and likelihood that adolescents in particular may not follow diet restrictions, relegate this to third-line status.

PEDIATRIC FDA INDICATIONS:
None.

ADULT FDA INDICATIONS:
Major depression.

OFF-LABEL USES:
Treatment-resistant depression; panic disorder; treatment-resistant anxiety disorders.

DOSAGE FORMS:
Transdermal patch: 6 mg, 9 mg, 12 mg/24 hours.

PEDIATRIC DOSAGE GUIDANCE:
- No dosing guidance in children and adolescents.
- Start 6 mg/24 hours QD; may ↑ in increments of 3 mg/24 hours every four weeks, up to max 12 mg/24 hours.
- Apply to clean, dry, intact skin on upper torso (below neck and above waist), upper thigh, or outer surface of upper arm; apply at the same time each day and rotate application sites; wash hands with soap and water after handling; avoid touching sticky side of patch.

MONITORING: No routine monitoring recommended unless clinical picture warrants.

COST: $$$$$

SIDE EFFECTS:
- Most common: Headache, insomnia, application site reaction, hypotension, diarrhea, dry mouth.
- Serious but rare: Orthostatic hypotension; caution in patients at risk (elderly, cerebrovascular disease, cardiovascular disease, hypovolemia).

MECHANISM, PHARMACOKINETICS, AND DRUG INTERACTIONS:
- Non-selective monoamine oxidase inhibitor.
- Metabolized primarily through CYP2B6 (also 2C9, 3A4/5) to active (N-desmethylselegiline, amphetamine, methamphetamine) and inactive metabolites; t ½: 18–25 hours.
- Avoid with other antidepressants, serotonergic agents, stimulants, sympathomimetics, dextromethorphan, disulfiram, meperidine, and carbamazepine. Do not use within five weeks of fluoxetine discontinuation or two weeks of other antidepressant discontinuation. Discontinue at least 10 days prior to elective surgery. Antihypertensives may exaggerate hypotensive effects. For doses higher than 6 mg, avoid use with foods or supplements high in tyramine, tryptophan, phenylalanine, or tyrosine.
- Wait two weeks after discontinuing transdermal selegiline before initiating therapy with serotonergic or any other contraindicated drug.

EVIDENCE AND CLINICAL PEARLS:
- Only one study in adolescents with depression, which showed that it was well tolerated but had no benefit over placebo.
- Oral selegiline (Eldepryl) used in Parkinson's disease (≤10 mg/day) is a selective inhibitor of MAO-B, which metabolizes dopamine. When used transdermally as EMSAM, selegiline achieves higher blood levels and non-selectively inhibits both MAO-A and MAO-B. Its antidepressant effect is thought to be due to its MAO-A inhibition, which blocks the breakdown of other centrally active neurotransmitters (norepinephrine, serotonin).
- When using 6 mg/day patch, no special diet required. When using higher doses, a tyramine-restricted diet should be followed.
- Patch may contain conducting metal (eg, aluminum); avoid exposure of application site to external heat source, which may increase the amount of drug absorbed.

FUN FACT:
Named "EMSAM" after Emily and Samuel, the children of the CEO of Somerset Pharmaceuticals (original manufacturer).

SERTRALINE (Zoloft) Fact Sheet [G]

BOTTOM LINE:
Consider sertraline a first-line agent for kids with depression and anxiety disorders.

PEDIATRIC FDA INDICATIONS:
OCD (6+ years).

ADULT FDA INDICATIONS:
Major depression; panic disorder; PTSD; PMDD; social anxiety.

OFF-LABEL USES:
Generalized anxiety disorder.

DOSAGE FORMS:
- **Tablets (G):** 25 mg (scored), 50 mg (scored), 100 mg (scored).
- **Capsules (G):** 150 mg, 200 mg.
- **Oral solution concentrate (G):** 20 mg/mL (must be diluted prior to administration).

PEDIATRIC DOSAGE GUIDANCE:
- Ages 6–12: Start 12.5–25 mg QD, increase by 25–50 mg/day increments weekly; max 200 mg/day.
- Ages 13–17: Start 25–50 mg QD, increase by 25–50 mg/day increments weekly; max 200 mg/day.
- Can be taken in the morning or night, depending on patient or family preference.

MONITORING: No routine monitoring recommended unless clinical picture warrants.

COST: $; capsule: $$$

SIDE EFFECTS:
- Most common: Nausea, insomnia, anxiety, apathy, headache.
- Serious but rare: Hyponatremia, mainly in the elderly; gastrointestinal bleeding, especially when combined with NSAIDs such as ibuprofen.

MECHANISM, PHARMACOKINETICS, AND DRUG INTERACTIONS:
- Selective serotonin reuptake inhibitor.
- Metabolized primarily through CYP2C19 (and to a lesser extent 2D6, 3A4); at higher doses (>150 mg/day), may moderately inhibit CYP2D6; t ½: 26 hours.
- Avoid use with MAOIs (allow a two-week washout period); avoid other serotonergic agents (serotonin syndrome).

EVIDENCE AND CLINICAL PEARLS:
- FDA approval for OCD in children is based on two positive trials. One was a 12-week randomized study of 112 kids ages 7–17 with OCD that found both CBT alone and sertraline alone to be significantly more effective than placebo, and the combination to be significantly more effective than either alone. The second was a 12-week randomized controlled trial of 187 kids (ages 6–18) that found sertraline was significantly more effective than placebo on all OCD outcome measures.
- Sertraline is also significantly more effective than placebo in children with depression based on a pooled analysis of two 10-week randomized studies of 364 patients (69% of sertraline vs 59% of placebo kids had >40% reduction of baseline symptoms).
- Generally, higher doses of SSRIs are required for treating OCD.
- Oral concentrate is formulated in 12% alcohol. Avoid use with disulfiram.

FUN FACT:
Zoloft is often remembered for the TV ad with the narration "You know when the world seems like a sad and lonely place?" An animated blob goes from shaky and isolated to happy; led by an orange butterfly, it bounces, smiles, and emerges from a cave to join two other blobs.

TRAZODONE Fact Sheet [G]

BOTTOM LINE:
Limited evidence to support its use, but fairly commonly used for insomnia in clinical practice.

PEDIATRIC FDA INDICATIONS:
None.

ADULT FDA INDICATIONS:
Major depression.

OFF-LABEL USES:
Insomnia; anxiety.

DOSAGE FORMS:
Tablets (G): 50 mg, 100 mg, 150 mg, 300 mg (scored).

PEDIATRIC DOSAGE GUIDANCE:
* Depression:
  – Ages 6–12: Start 1.5–2 mg/kg/day divided TID; ↑ every three to four days to response; max 6 mg/kg/day.
  – Ages 13–17: Start 25 mg BID–TID, increase dose every three to four days; max dose 6 mg/kg/day up to 400 mg/day.
* Insomnia (off label): Start 25 mg QHS; may ↑ by 25 mg increments every two weeks, up to 200 mg QHS.
* Generally best given at bedtime, though some patients find the medication stimulating and need to take it in the morning.

MONITORING: No routine monitoring recommended unless clinical picture warrants.

COST: $

SIDE EFFECTS:
* Most common: Drowsiness, dry mouth, dizziness or lightheadedness, orthostatic hypotension, headache, blurred vision, nausea, or vomiting.
* Serious but rare: Reports of priapism (painful erection >6 hours in duration); may require surgical or pharmacologic (eg, epinephrine) intervention and may result in impotence or permanent impairment of erectile function. Orthostatic hypotension and syncope reported (less at hypnotic doses).

MECHANISM, PHARMACOKINETICS, AND DRUG INTERACTIONS:
* Serotonin reuptake inhibitor, alpha-1 adrenergic receptor antagonist, and serotonin 5HT2A and 5HT2C receptor antagonist.
* Metabolized primarily through CYP3A4 to active metabolite (mCPP), which in turn is metabolized by 2D6; induces P-glycoprotein; t ½: 7–10 hours.
* Avoid use with MAOIs.

EVIDENCE AND CLINICAL PEARLS:
* Although efficacy data in kids are lacking, fairly commonly used to manage sleep in kids.
* If daytime drowsiness occurs, administer the majority of dosage at bedtime or ↓ dose.
* Trazodone's hypnotic effects are not due to anticholinergic or antihistaminergic effects.
* IR formulation rarely used as antidepressant due to risk for oversedation and orthostasis at therapeutic doses; majority of IR use currently is for insomnia.

FUN FACT:
As a consequence of the production of mCPP as a metabolite, patients taking trazodone may test positive on urine tests for the presence of MDMA (ecstasy).

TRICYCLIC ANTIDEPRESSANTS (TCAs) Fact Sheet [G]

BOTTOM LINE:
Not commonly used due to side effects and toxicity risk; however, TCAs should be considered for kids who do not respond to other antidepressants.

PEDIATRIC FDA INDICATIONS:
OCD (clomipramine, 10–17 years); **nocturnal enuresis** (imipramine, 6–17 years).

ADULT FDA INDICATIONS:
Major depression; OCD.

OFF-LABEL USES:
Headache; migraine; neuropathic pain; fibromyalgia; anxiety disorders; insomnia; cataplexy; sleep terrors; sleepwalking.

Note: Nine TCAs are FDA approved for adult use in depression (amitriptyline, amoxapine, desipramine, doxepin, imipramine, maprotiline, nortriptyline, protriptyline, trimipramine) and one is approved for OCD (clomipramine). We've selected the ones most commonly used in kids.

DOSAGE FORMS:
- **Amitriptyline tablets (G):** 10 mg, 25 mg, 50 mg, 75 mg, 100 mg, 150 mg.
- **Clomipramine capsules (Anafranil, [G]):** 25 mg, 50 mg, 75 mg.
- **Desipramine tablets (Norpramin, [G]):** 10 mg, 25 mg, 50 mg, 75 mg, 100 mg, 150 mg.
- **Imipramine tablets and capsules (G):** 10 mg, 25 mg, 50 mg, 75 mg, 100 mg, 125 mg, 150 mg.
- **Nortriptyline capsules (Pamelor, [G]):** 10 mg, 25 mg, 50 mg, 75 mg, and 10 mg/5 mL oral solution.

PEDIATRIC DOSAGE GUIDANCE:
- Amitriptyline or imipramine: For ages 6–12, start 1 mg/kg/day divided TID, increase by 0.5 mg/kg/day every three days; max 5 mg/kg/day or 200 mg/day. For ages 3–17, start 25–50 mg QHS or divided TID, ↑ by 10–25 mg/day intervals every three days; max 200 mg/day.
- Clomipramine: Start 25 mg QHS and ↑ by 25 mg/day every four to seven days; max 200 mg/day.
- Desipramine: Start 25 mg QHS, ↑ by 25 mg/day intervals every four to seven days; max 150 mg/day.
- Nortriptyline: For ages 6–12, start 1 mg/kg/day divided TID, increase by 0.5 mg/kg/day every three days; max 150 mg/day. For ages 13–17, start 25–50 mg QHS or divided TID, ↑ by 10–50 mg/day intervals every three days; max 150 mg/day.
- For enuresis: Imipramine 10 mg QHS, increase by 10 mg/day increments every one to two weeks; max 75 mg/day.

MONITORING: ECG in patients at risk.

COST: Clomipramine: $$; all others: $

SIDE EFFECTS:
- Most common: Sedation, dry mouth, constipation, weight gain, sexual side effects, urinary hesitation, blurred vision.
- Serious but rare: Seizure; cardiac effects including orthostasis, arrhythmias, QT prolongation, AV block.

MECHANISM, PHARMACOKINETICS, AND DRUG INTERACTIONS:
- Serotonin and norepinephrine reuptake inhibitor.
- Metabolized primarily through liver, likely CYP2D6 primarily; t ½: 18–44 hours.
- Avoid use with other serotonergic antidepressants or agents with hypotensive or anticholinergic effects.

EVIDENCE AND CLINICAL PEARLS:
- Only one small study (n = 30), of nearly a dozen placebo-controlled studies of TCAs in children and adolescents, showed positive results. A meta-analysis similarly found no efficacy for depression in kids.
- Nortriptyline improved symptoms of ADHD in kids, but the effect was not as robust as with stimulants.
- Clomipramine can be very effective in childhood OCD but has a greater side effect burden.
- TCAs reduce frequency of bedwetting in kids with enuresis, but benefits are not sustained after medication is discontinued. Behavioral interventions and alarms are preferred.
- Divided doses (BID–TID) may help with tolerability initially; convert to QHS to minimize daytime sedation.
- Overdose toxicity with potentially serious cardiac effects or fatality with as little as 10-day supply. Sudden death reported in several patients taking therapeutic doses of TCAs. Avoid use in those at risk.

FUN FACT:
Imipramine was the first antidepressant approved in the US, developed by tweaking the molecular structure of the antipsychotic Thorazine. It didn't work for psychosis, but was the first wonder drug for depression and anxiety.

VENLAFAXINE (Effexor, Effexor XR) Fact Sheet [G]

BOTTOM LINE:
Fewer data than SSRIs places venlafaxine in the second-line category for both depression and GAD in kids.

PEDIATRIC FDA INDICATIONS:
None.

ADULT FDA INDICATIONS:
Major depression; social anxiety disorder; GAD; panic disorder.

OFF-LABEL USES:
PTSD; PMDD; vasomotor symptoms of menopause; diabetic peripheral neuropathy; fibromyalgia.

DOSAGE FORMS:
- **Tablets (G):** 25 mg, 37.5 mg, 50 mg, 75 mg, 100 mg (scored).
- **ER tablets (G):** 37.5 mg, 75 mg, 150 mg, 225 mg.

PEDIATRIC DOSAGE GUIDANCE:
- Depression:
  – Ages 8–12: Start 12.5 mg QD or 37.5 mg as XR once daily; ↑ dose by 12.5 mg/day (IR) or 37.5 mg/day (XR) increments at intervals of four or more days; max 75 mg/day (divided TID for IR). IR may be switched to nearest equivalent daily dose of XR QD.
  – Ages 13–17: Start 25 mg QD or 37.5 mg as XR QD, ↑ dose by 25 mg/day (IR) or 37.5 mg/day (XR) increments at intervals of four or more days; max 75 mg/day (divided TID for IR). ER max dose 225 mg/day in adolescents.
- Anxiety:
  – XR: Start 37.5 mg QD, ↑ by 37.5 mg/day at weekly intervals; max 225 mg/day.

MONITORING: Periodic BP.

COST: $

SIDE EFFECTS:
- Most common: Anorexia, constipation, dizziness, dry mouth, nausea, nervousness, somnolence, sweating, sexual side effects, headache, insomnia.
- Serious but rare: Sustained, dose-related hypertension reported. May cause hyponatremia or SIADH; use with caution in patients who are volume-depleted, elderly, or taking diuretics.

MECHANISM, PHARMACOKINETICS, AND DRUG INTERACTIONS:
- Serotonin and norepinephrine reuptake inhibitor.
- Metabolized primarily through CYP2D6 to O-desmethylvenlafaxine (ODV), major active metabolite (an SNRI, marketed as Pristiq), and also by CYP3A4; inhibitor of CYP2D6; t ½: 5 hours (11 hours for ODV).
- Avoid use with MAOIs and other serotonergic agents. Caution with CYP2D6 or 3A4 inhibitors, which may increase venlafaxine levels.

EVIDENCE AND CLINICAL PEARLS
- An open study suggested venlafaxine may be effective for adolescent depression, but two randomized controlled studies in kids (7–17 years) with depression found venlafaxine was no better than placebo.
- Two randomized double-blind placebo-controlled studies in more than 300 children and adolescents with GAD showed greater improvement with venlafaxine compared to placebo. Efficacy has been shown in social phobia as well.
- For patients with nausea, start at lower dose, titrate more slowly, and give with food.
- May cause false positive for PCP in a urine drug screen.
- Increase in blood pressure much more likely in doses >225 mg/day.
- Significant discontinuation syndrome, even with XR formulation. Taper by no more than 75 mg/week to discontinue.

FUN FACT:
Venlafaxine is structurally related to the atypical opioid analgesic tramadol (Ultram), itself a serotonergic agent, but not to any other antidepressant drugs.

Antipsychotics

Antipsychotics are potent medications that have been likened to chemotherapy for the brain. Their use in children and adolescents can yield impressive results, but they can also lead to very problematic side effects. It is important to stay current on research trends and take clinical situations one at a time. Try not to be swayed by occasional cases of spectacular improvement or extreme side effects. Document your rationale, including possible risks and benefits. Most importantly, advocate for comprehensive care, which can reduce the need for these medications and their attendant risks.

Here are some tips on using antipsychotics in children and adolescents.

EFFICACY

Antipsychotics have many uses, both on and off label. They are FDA approved (marked by an *) or have some evidence supporting use for the following indications in children and adolescents:

- Positive and negative psychotic symptoms*
- Irritability in autism*
- Bipolar disorder, including depression and mood instability*
- Augmentation of antidepressants*
- Tourette's disorder*
- Augmentation for treatment-resistant OCD
- Second- or third-line treatment for situations involving aggression

There are also many off-label uses for antipsychotics. They may benefit patients with borderline personality traits, eating disorders, and PTSD, usually in small doses. Early indications for chlorpromazine included such nonspecific symptoms as hyperactivity, agitation, anxiety, and "severe behavior," perhaps contributing to overreliance on this entire class of medications. While antipsychotics can be quite helpful, it's important to remember that they cannot make up for a lack of good therapy or cover for an absence of adult supervision.

Neurotoxicity and Mortality

Research is growing on neurotoxicity and mortality associated with antipsychotic medications. Brain volume change and cortical thinning is seen in adolescents and young adults with schizophrenia. The loss of brain volume is more pronounced depending on illness duration, disease severity, substance use (particularly alcohol and cannabis), and antipsychotic dosage. Mortality rates are nearly 80% higher in children and adolescents treated with high-dose antipsychotics. Moreover, antipsychotics are not particularly effective for many of their off-label uses, such as severe ADHD or efforts to reduce the frequency of seclusion or restraint. For these reasons alone, we recommend using these medications conservatively and reducing or discontinuing them when possible.

CHOOSING ANTIPSYCHOTICS

With all the options available, it can be difficult to decide which antipsychotic to prescribe.

We avoid first-generation antipsychotics with their higher risk of extrapyramidal symptoms (EPS). We steer clear of newer second-generation antipsychotics with fewer safety studies. We favor olanzapine, quetiapine, risperidone, aripiprazole, ziprasidone, and lurasidone, choosing specific medications based on side effects. If we want to avoid sedation and hunger, we might opt for lurasidone or ziprasidone. If a person needs to sleep and eat, we might try olanzapine or quetiapine. Risperidone and aripiprazole often have more research to support efficacy, eg, with autism. For treatment-resistant patients, clozapine (off label) is probably underutilized. These are rough guidelines as individuals will respond differently.

While new antipsychotics typically come with promises of fewer side effects, we never know much about the real risks until medications have been on the market for many years. One study reported that in a third of FDA-approved medications, new side effects became apparent only after the agents were approved. Also, many of the recent studies of second-generation antipsychotics are conducted by the drug companies, which have a history of misrepresenting data. If you decide to try a new medication, be sure to include consideration of unknown risks as part of your ongoing process of informed consent.

DISCONTINUING ANTIPSYCHOTICS

When a person responds well to an antipsychotic, we may be tempted to keep it going and make the most of its efficacy, even though there may be substantial side effects and little evidence to support chronic use. For instance, in autism we do not have data for efficacy beyond six months. On the other hand, we often feel pressed to wean the person off the medication to reduce side effects, but discontinuation often leads to relapse, and relapse often makes recapture of symptoms more difficult. Your chances of success in reducing or discontinuing medication will relate in large part to how well the patient is doing at home, at school, and in the community; whether good psychosocial supports are in place; and whether there are big changes coming in the near term (eg, divorce, school changes, a major move). We recommend that you plan to do a gradual discontinuation at some point, and to go as slowly as practically possible when weaning. If you later need to return to prior levels and continue to live with the risks, at least you will have evidence that the medication is helping.

SIDE EFFECTS

1. **EPS.** For antipsychotics, these include dystonia, akathisia, and Parkinsonism. Dystonic reactions are painful and frightening. They might include torticollis (twisting neck), opisthotonos (arching back), or oculogyric crisis (eyes rolled back). Tongue swelling can block the airway, causing choking when eating and potentially aspiration pneumonia. Akathisia—severe internal restlessness—can look like overactivity and can create overwhelming anxiety and even suicidality. You may need to use anticholinergics such as benztropine for dystonia or beta-blockers such as propranolol for akathisia. Some patients benefit from very early use of these. We suggest reviewing EPS as part of informed consent. Although it is rare, you should review the risk of neuroleptic malignant syndrome, which is a potentially life-threatening form of catatonia. If a patient becomes hot, with stiff muscles, perhaps with agitation and/or confusion, they need to have an immediate assessment at an emergency department. Do a formal screen for signs of tardive dyskinesia (TD) at least every six months, eg, with an Abnormal Involuntary Movement Scale (AIMS). (You will find information on conducting the AIMS in the appendices.) Some kids can't cooperate with an AIMS, so you will need to document whatever you are able to see in the office, and perhaps ask parents for home videos if they are reporting new abnormal movements.

2. **Metabolic changes.** Your skinny, out-of-control patient can bloom into a heavy and perhaps still out-of-control patient in a few months. Some people become clinically worse due to their ravenous appetite caused by the medication, becoming more disruptive or devious in their hunt for food. Diet and exercise can be critically important. Choose medications with less propensity for weight gain when you can, and think about starting metformin along with the medication since current research shows that it works to prevent weight gain on antipsychotics in children and adolescents but does little to help once the patient has already gained the weight. Stimulants and topiramate have been tried to mitigate weight gain, although these are also off-label uses. Stimulants have not been shown to help, and topiramate works better before the weight gain has occurred—like metformin, but less effective. Consider using GLP-1 agonists to prevent weight gain on antipsychotics for patients who are already at a BMI of 30 or higher. Regular metabolic checks are important, including weight and height, calculation of BMI, fasting lipids and glucose, and perhaps HbA1c and prolactin (with risperidone). Also track waist circumference in adult-sized patients. Women with a waist of 35 inches or greater and men with a waist of 40 inches or greater are at higher risk of type 2 diabetes and cardiovascular disease. Another similar parameter is a waist-to-height ratio of greater than 0.5. Check labs and physical parameters before treatment, and if they remain normal, at one, three, and six months, then annually. Note that weight gain can also lead to more rapid onset of puberty, with early appearance of secondary sex characteristics and premature closure of growth plates with shorter stature. Early puberty places this already vulnerable population of children at an even greater risk for depression and anxiety in their adolescence. Perhaps most important, we need to be mindful to address the potentially severe psychological impacts of weight such as fat shaming and other kinds of weight-based bias.

TABLE 4: Pediatric Metabolic Monitoring Parameters With Antipsychotic Medications

	Baseline	Week 4	Week 8	Week 12	Every 3 Months	Every 6–12 Months
Height, weight, BMI	X	X	X	X	X	X
Blood pressure/pulse	X			X		X
Fasting glucose, HbA1c	X			X		X
Fasting lipids	X			X		X

3. **Cardiac issues.** Antipsychotics can sometimes create or exacerbate arrhythmias, including QT prolongation with risk for torsades de pointes. Get a good cardiac history and family medical history before starting these medications and consider ordering a screening ECG if there is a significant history of cardiac disease. Some antipsychotics, particularly first-generation ones such as chlorpromazine, can also cause orthostatic hypotension.

4. **Prolactin issues.** Some antipsychotics may increase prolactin levels, potentially affecting onset of puberty. Risperidone poses the greatest risk, whereas aripiprazole may have the lowest risk. In patients who present with gynecomastia, prolactin level should be checked. Prolactinemia should also be considered in patients who present with menstrual changes or delayed onset of menarche.

CLASS WARNINGS

All of the second-generation antipsychotics carry the same FDA class warnings. Rather than repeating all of these concerns on each fact sheet, we will mention the warnings here. Some of these are specific to the geriatric population, but we are including them here for completeness.

- In 2003, the FDA required all manufacturers of second-generation antipsychotics to revise their package labeling to reflect the potential risks for weight gain, hyperglycemia, new-onset or worsening diabetes, and hyperlipidemias. While this has become a class warning, it's clear that there are a handful of really bad actors here: Clozapine and olanzapine are the worst, aripiprazole and risperidone relatively less so, and lurasidone and ziprasidone the least likely offenders.

- Patient-specific factors may also play a role. In general, the incidence and severity of weight gain and metabolic effects appear to be greater in the pediatric population.

- A black box warning for all agents in this class suggests a substantially **higher mortality rate in geriatric patients with dementia-related psychosis** receiving second-generation antipsychotics (4.5%) compared with those receiving placebo (2.6%). Although most fatalities resulted from cardiac-related events (eg, heart failure, sudden death) or infections (mostly pneumonia) as opposed to a clearly direct effect of medication, second-generation antipsychotics are *not* approved for the treatment of dementia-related psychosis, and such use should be avoided or minimized when possible.

- **Adverse cerebrovascular events** (eg, stroke, TIA), sometimes fatal, have been reported in geriatric patients (73–97 years of age) with dementia-related psychosis. The FDA has issued a black box warning on second-generation antipsychotics to reflect this risk; several studies have shown that cerebrovascular event risk is elevated with first-generation antipsychotics as well.

- **Neuroleptic malignant syndrome, a form of malignant catatonia,** is a potentially fatal syndrome that has been reported in patients receiving antipsychotic agents. It is characterized by fever, severe muscle rigidity, and autonomic instability. Treatment requires immediate discontinuation of the drug and intensive symptomatic treatment in a hospital setting, often use of high dosages of lorazepam, and perhaps ECT as a life-saving procedure (see the next chapter on Anxiolytics and Hypnotics as well as the catatonia algorithm in that chapter).

Antipsychotics

Psychosis Treatment Algorithm for Children and Adolescents

*Denotes off label

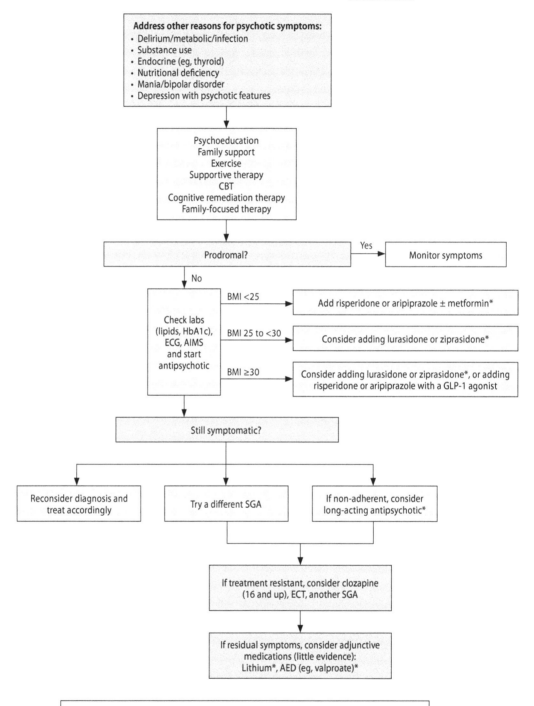

Address other reasons for psychotic symptoms:
- Delirium/metabolic/infection
- Substance use
- Endocrine (eg, thyroid)
- Nutritional deficiency
- Mania/bipolar disorder
- Depression with psychotic features

↓

Psychoeducation
Family support
Exercise
Supportive therapy
CBT
Cognitive remediation therapy
Family-focused therapy

↓

Prodromal? —— Yes → Monitor symptoms

↓ No

Check labs (lipids, HbA1c), ECG, AIMS and start antipsychotic

- BMI <25 → Add risperidone or aripiprazole ± metformin*
- BMI 25 to <30 → Consider adding lurasidone or ziprasidone*
- BMI ≥30 → Consider adding lurasidone or ziprasidone*, or adding risperidone or aripiprazole with a GLP-1 agonist

↓

Still symptomatic?

- Reconsider diagnosis and treat accordingly
- Try a different SGA
- If non-adherent, consider long-acting antipsychotic*

↓

If treatment resistant, consider clozapine (16 and up), ECT, another SGA

↓

If residual symptoms, consider adjunctive medications (little evidence):
Lithium*, AED (eg, valproate)*

- Use non-pharmacologic approaches first when possible to help reduce use of medication
- See text and tables for specific age-related guidance
- If using antipsychotics, check weight and labs (lipids, HbA1c, others as indicated) at baseline, 12 weeks, and yearly or sooner, AIMS at baseline and every 6 months or sooner, and consider ECG at baseline and yearly or sooner
- If stable for 6 months, consider gradual taper and discontinuation of medications

Autism Support Treatment Algorithm for Children and Adolescents

*Denotes off label

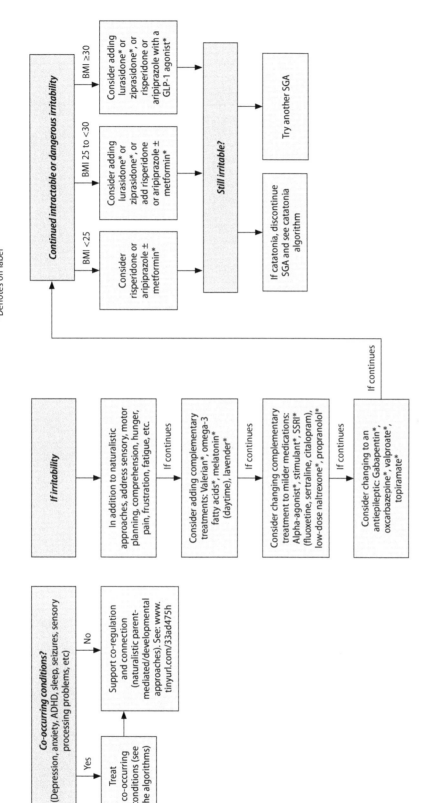

Co-occurring conditions?
(Depression, anxiety, ADHD, sleep, seizures, sensory processing problems, etc)

- **Yes** → Treat co-occurring conditions (see the algorithms)
- **No** → Support co-regulation and connection (naturalistic parent-mediated/developmental approaches). See: www.tinyurl.com/33ad475h

If irritability

→ In addition to naturalistic approaches, address sensory, motor planning, comprehension, hunger, pain, frustration, fatigue, etc.

If continues

→ Consider adding complementary treatments: Valerian*, omega-3 fatty acids*, melatonin* (daytime), lavender*

If continues

→ Consider changing complementary treatment to milder medications: Alpha-agonist*, stimulant*, SSRI* (fluoxetine, sertraline, citalopram), low-dose naltrexone*, propranolol*

If continues

→ Consider changing to an antiepileptic: Gabapentin*, oxcarbazepine*, valproate*, topiramate*

If continues →

Continued intractable or dangerous irritability

- **BMI <25** → Consider risperidone or aripiprazole ± metformin*
- **BMI 25 to <30** → Consider adding lurasidone* or ziprasidone*, or add risperidone or aripiprazole ± metformin*
- **BMI ≥30** → Consider adding lurasidone* or ziprasidone*, or risperidone or aripiprazole with a GLP-1 agonist*

Still irritable?

→ Try another SGA

→ If catatonia, discontinue SGA and see catatonia algorithm

- Use non-pharmacologic approaches first when possible to help reduce use of medication
- See text and tables for specific age-related guidance
- If using antidepressants, discuss potential side effects including rare but possible increase in behavioral activation or suicidal thinking
- If using antipsychotics, check weight and labs (lipids, HbA1c, others as indicated) at baseline, 12 weeks, and yearly or sooner, AIMS at baseline and every 6 months or sooner, and consider ECG at baseline and yearly or sooner
- If stable for 3–6 months, consider gradual taper and discontinuation of medications

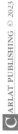

ARLAT PUBLISHING © 2023

Antipsychotics

TABLE 5: First-Generation Antipsychotics

Generic Name (Brand Name) Year FDA Approved [G] denotes generic availability	Relevant FDA Indication(s) (Pediatric indications in bold)	Available Strengths (mg)	Dosage Equivalents	Usual Pediatric Dosage Range (starting–max) (mg)	EPS and Akathisia	Anticholinergic	Relative Sedation and Orthostasis	Notes
Chlorpromazine [G] (Thorazine[1]) 1957	Psychosis, mania, **nausea/ vomiting; severe behavioral problems (0.5–17); excessive motor activity**	Tablet: 10, 25, 50, 100, 200 Liquid: 30 mg/mL, 100 mg/mL IM: 25 mg/mL	100	10–200	Low	Moderate	High	Injectable available; photosensitivity
Haloperidol [G] (Haldol, Haldol Decanoate) 1967	**Psychosis (3–17), Tourette's disorder (3–17), severe behavioral problems (3–17); excessive motor activity**	Tablet: 0.5, 1, 2, 5, 10, 20 Liquid: 2 mg/mL IM: 2 mg/mL LAI: See LAI table	2	0.25–10	Very high	Low	Low	Oral solution; injectables (short and LAI) available
Perphenazine [G] (Trilafon[1]) 1957	**Schizophrenia (12 and older);** severe nausea/ vomiting	Tablet: 2, 4, 8, 16	8	8–64	High	Low	Low	Insufficient evidence in kids; mid-potency agent with lower EPS potential than haloperidol

[1]Brand discontinued; no longer available as brand

TABLE 6: Second-Generation Antipsychotics

Generic Name (Brand Name) Year FDA Approved [G] denotes generic availability	Relevant FDA Indication(s) (Pediatric indications in bold)	Available Strengths (mg)	Usual Pediatric Dosage Range (starting–max) (mg)[1]	Weight Gain and Metabolic Effects[2]	EPS and Akathisia	QT Prolongation	Notes
Aripiprazole [G] (Abilify, Abilify Discmelt) 2002	**Schizophrenia (13+)** **Bipolar mania, monotherapy and adjunctive (10+)** Bipolar maintenance, monotherapy and adjunctive; Depression adjunct; **Irritability in autism (6–17)** **Tourette's disorder (6–18)** Agitation in schizophrenia or bipolar (IM only); Acute schizophrenia relapse (LAI only)	Tablet: 2, 5, 10, 15, 20, 30; ODT: 10, 15, 20, 30; Liquid: 1 mg/mL; LAI: See LAI fact sheet and table	2–30 QD	Moderate	High (mainly akathisia)	Low	Can be "activating"
Asenapine (Saphris) 2009	Schizophrenia; **Bipolar mania, monotherapy and adjunctive (10+)**	Tablet: 2.5, 5, 10 (sublingual only); Patch: 3.8, 5.7, 7.6/24 hrs	SL: 5–10 BID; TD: 3.8–7.6 QD	Moderate	Moderate	Low	Avoid food or drink for 10 minutes after taking; sedating
Brexpiprazole (Rexulti) 2015	**Schizophrenia (13+)** Depression adjunct	Tablet: 0.25, 0.5, 1, 2, 3, 4	0.5–4 QD	Moderate	High (mainly akathisia)	Low	Newer agent with limited data in kids
Clozapine [G] (Clozaril, FazaClo, Versacloz) 1989 Generic not available for oral suspension	Treatment-resistant schizophrenia; Recurrent suicidal behavior in schizophrenia or schizoaffective disorders	Tablet: 25, 50, 100, 200; ODT: 12.5, 25, 100, 150, 200; Oral suspension: 50 mg/mL	12.5–450 BID	High	Low	Low	Probably most effective AP, though data in kids limited
Lurasidone (Latuda) 2010	**Schizophrenia (13+)** **Bipolar I depression (10+)**	Tablet: 20, 40, 60, 80, 120	40–80 QD	Moderate	Moderate	Low	Sedating; must take with food
Olanzapine [G] (Zyprexa, Zyprexa Zydis) 1996 Generic not available for LAI	**Schizophrenia (13+)** **Bipolar mania, monotherapy and adjunctive (13+)** Bipolar maintenance, monotherapy; Agitation in schizophrenia or bipolar (IM only); **Bipolar I depression in combination with fluoxetine (10+)** Treatment-resistant depression in combination with fluoxetine	Tablet: 2.5, 5, 7.5, 10, 15, 20; ODT: 5, 10, 15, 20; IM injection: 10 mg/vial; LAI: See LAI fact sheet and table	2.5–20 QD	High	Low/moderate	Low	Greatest weight gain, metabolic effects; somnolence
Olanzapine/samidorphan (Lybalvi) 2021	Schizophrenia; Bipolar mania, monotherapy and adjunctive; Bipolar maintenance	Tablet: 5/10, 10/10, 15/10, 20/10	5/10–20/10 QD	Moderate	Low/moderate	Low	Less weight gain but still moderate risk; avoid opioids

Antipsychotics

Generic Name (Brand Name) Year FDA Approved [G] denotes generic availability	Relevant FDA Indication(s) (Pediatric indications in bold)	Available Strengths (mg)	Usual Pediatric Dosage Range (starting–max) (mg)[1]	Weight Gain and Metabolic Effects[2]	EPS and Akathisia	QT Prolongation	Notes
Paliperidone [G] (Invega) 2006 Generic not available for LAI	**Schizophrenia (12+)** Schizoaffective disorder	ER tablet: 1.5, 3, 6, 9 LAI: See LAI fact sheet and table	3–12 QD	Moderate	High	Moderate	Good for those with hepatic impairment; increases prolactin; fewer data in kids than risperidone
Quetiapine [G] (Seroquel, Seroquel XR) 1997	**Schizophrenia (13+)** **Bipolar mania, monotherapy and adjunctive (10+)** Bipolar maintenance Bipolar I or II depression Depression adjunct (ER formulation)	Tablet: 25, 50, 100, 200, 300, 400 ER tablet: 50, 150, 200, 300, 400	50–800 daily, divided BID to TID; 300–800 QHS for XR	Moderate	Low	Moderate	Sedating; weight gain
Risperidone [G] (Risperdal, Risperdal M-Tab) 1993 Generic not available for LAI	**Schizophrenia (13+)** **Bipolar mania, monotherapy and adjunctive (10+)** **Irritability in autism (5–17)**	Tablet: 0.25, 0.5, 1, 2, 3, 4 ODT: 0.25, 0.5, 1, 2, 3, 4 LAI: See LAI fact sheet and table	0.5–6 divided QD to BID	Moderate	High	Low	Increases prolactin; often produces EPS; weight gain
Ziprasidone [G] (Geodon) 2001	Schizophrenia Bipolar mania, monotherapy Bipolar maintenance, adjunctive Agitation in schizophrenia (IM injection)	Capsule: 20, 40, 60, 80 IM injection: 20 mg/mL	20–80 BID	Low–moderate	Low	High	Take with food; limited data in kids; increases prolactin; EPS; weight gain

ODT = orally disintegrating tablet; LAI = long-acting injectable; ER, XR = extended release

[1] For schizophrenia indication

[2] Significant weight gain and metabolic symptoms may occur in kids even with lower-risk agents

TABLE 7: Comparison of Relative Side Effects Among Antipsychotics

	Wt/Metabolic	Sedation	QT Prolongation	Orthostasis	Akathisia	EPS (Park/Dyst)	TD	Prolactin	Anticholinergic	Seizures
First Generation										
Chlorpromazine	+	+++	++++	+++	+	+	+++	+	+++	++
Fluphenazine	+	+	++	+	+++	+++	+++	+++	+	+
Haloperidol	+	+	++	+	+++	+++	+++	+++	+	+
Loxapine	+	++	++	++	++	++	++	++	++	+
Molindone	0/+	++	++	+	++	++	++	++	+	+
Perphenazine	+	++	++	++	++	++	++	++	++	+
Thioridazine	+	+++	++++	+++	+	+	++	++	+++	++
Thiothixene	+	+	++	+	+++	+++	+++	+++	+	+++
Trifluoperazine	+	+	++	+	++	++	++	++	++	+
Second Generation										
Aripiprazole	++	+	0/+	+	+++	+	+	+	+	+
Asenapine	++	++	++	++	++	+	++	++	+	+
Brexpiprazole	++[1]	+	++	+	+++	+	+	+	+	+
Cariprazine	++	++	++	+	++	+	+	+	++	+
Clozapine	+++	+++	++	+++	0/+	0/+	0/+	+	+++	+++
Iloperidone	++	++	+++	+++	+	+	+	++	+	+
Lumateperone	+	+	+	++	+	+	+	+	+	+
Lurasidone	+	++	+	+	++	++	++	+	+	+
Olanzapine	+++	+++	++	++	++	++	+	++	++	++
Olanzapine/samidorphan	++	+++	++	++	++	++	+	++	++	++
Paliperidone	++	+	++	++	++	++	++	+++	+	+
Pimavanserin (Parkinson's psychosis only)	+	+	++	+	0	0	0	0	0	+
Quetiapine	++	+++	++	++	0/+	0/+	+	+	++	++
Risperidone	++	++	++	++	++	++	++	+++	+	+
Ziprasidone	0/+	++	+++	++	++	+	+	++	+	+

Adapted from *The American Psychiatric Association Practice Guideline for the Treatment of Patients With Schizophrenia, Third Edition* (September 2020) and based on adult data where pediatric data lacking

[1]Fewer data but similar to aripiprazole

Antipsychotics

ARIPIPRAZOLE (Abilify) Fact Sheet [G]

BOTTOM LINE:
Not as good a choice as we used to think for minimizing risk of weight gain and metabolic side effects, and beware of akathisia. Large number of indications and reports of success at a variety of doses make it difficult to predict dosing for individual patients.

PEDIATRIC FDA INDICATIONS:
Schizophrenia (13–17 years); **bipolar disorder,** acute treatment of manic and mixed episodes (10–17 years); **irritability in autism** (6–17 years); **Tourette's disorder** (6–18 years).

ADULT FDA INDICATIONS:
Schizophrenia; bipolar disorder, acute treatment of manic and mixed episodes; bipolar disorder, maintenance treatment; major depression, as adjunct.

OFF-LABEL USES:
Bipolar depression; behavioral disturbances.

DOSAGE FORMS:
- **Tablets (G):** 2 mg, 5 mg, 10 mg, 15 mg, 20 mg, 30 mg.
- **Orally disintegrating tablets (G):** 10 mg, 15 mg, 20 mg, 30 mg.
- **Oral liquid (G):** 1 mg/mL.
- **IM long-acting injectable:** Abilify Maintena: 300 mg and 400 mg; Aristada: 441 mg, 662 mg, 882 mg, 1064 mg; Aristada Initio: 675 mg (see LAI fact sheet and table).

PEDIATRIC DOSAGE GUIDANCE:
- Schizophrenia and bipolar disorder: Start 2 mg/day, increase on third day to 5 mg/day; may increase further by 5 mg/day increments weekly to target dose 10 mg/day, max 15 mg/day (<11 years) or 30 mg/day (≥12 years).
- Irritability in autism: Start 2 mg/day, increase up to 5 mg/day in weekly increments to target dose 5–10 mg/day, max 15 mg/day.
- Tourette's: Start 2 mg/day. For children <50 kg, ↑ to target 5 mg/day, max 10 mg/day. For children >50 kg, ↑ to target 10 mg/day, max 20 mg/day.
- Liquid dosing: Oral solution equivalent to tablet dose up to 25 mg; for 30 mg tablets, give 25 mg oral solution.
- Orally disintegrating tablet: Same as regular tablet dosing.

MONITORING: Weight, waist circumference, glucose, lipids, prolactin if symptoms, abnormal movements.

COST: $; liquid: $$$; ODT: $$$$

SIDE EFFECTS:
- Most common: Akathisia, anxiety, insomnia, sedation, tremors, EPS, weight gain.
- Serious but rare: Rare reports of pathologic gambling and other impulse control problems (eg, eating).

MECHANISM, PHARMACOKINETICS, AND DRUG INTERACTIONS:
- Dopamine D2 and serotonin 5HT1A receptor partial agonist and serotonin 5HT2A receptor antagonist.
- Metabolized by CYP2D6 and 3A4; t ½: 3–6 days.
- Use ½ usual dose in presence of 2D6 or 3A4 inhibitors or in known 2D6 poor metabolizers; ¼ dose if both 2D6 inhibitor/poor metabolizer and 3A4 inhibitor; double dose if also using 3A4 inducer.

EVIDENCE AND CLINICAL PEARLS:
- A 52-week randomized controlled trial of 146 adolescents with schizophrenia found a longer time to exacerbation of psychotic symptoms and relapse with aripiprazole compared with placebo.
- Aripiprazole is commonly used longer term in autism, despite lack of evidence for continued effectiveness.
- One four-week (n = 296) and one six-week trial (n = 43) compared aripiprazole with placebo in children with bipolar disorder (and comorbid ADHD in latter study) and found aripiprazole significantly more effective for mania than placebo.
- Two eight-week randomized trials in a total of 308 children (ages 6–17) with autism and irritability showed significant benefit with aripiprazole compared to placebo. In one continuation trial of 85 aripiprazole responders who were randomized to either continue aripiprazole or switch to placebo, no difference in time to relapse was seen.
- Several studies have demonstrated aripiprazole's efficacy in reducing tics in children with Tourette's disorder (significantly more than placebo, as well as equal to risperidone or haloperidol).
- One of two FDA-approved medications for irritability in autism. Also, some prescribers use low-dose aripiprazole to counteract antipsychotic-induced prolactinemia, given its partial agonist properties.

FUN FACT:
After aripiprazole's generic launch, Otsuka followed up with brexpiprazole, another dopamine partial agonist, approved for use in adults with schizophrenia and depression (as adjunct) and now in clinical trials for ADHD.

ASENAPINE (Saphris, Secuado) Fact Sheet [G]

BOTTOM LINE:
Since there are no clear advantages over other second-generation antipsychotics and minimal evidence for efficacy in children, the only reason to prescribe Saphris or Secuado is if your patient can't or doesn't want to swallow a pill. Mouth numbness, sedation, dizziness, akathisia, weight gain, and potential for allergic reaction are significant liabilities with the former and skin irritation with the latter. Not recommended for first-line use.

PEDIATRIC FDA INDICATIONS:
Bipolar disorder, acute monotherapy treatment of manic or mixed episodes (10–17 years); SL formulation only.

ADULT FDA INDICATIONS:
Schizophrenia; bipolar disorder, acute and maintenance treatment of manic or mixed episodes.

OFF-LABEL USES:
Bipolar maintenance; bipolar depression; behavioral disturbances; impulse control disorders.

DOSAGE FORMS:
• **SL tablets (G):** 2.5 mg, 5 mg, 10 mg.
• **Transdermal patch (Secuado):** 3.8 mg, 5.7 mg, 7.6 mg/24 hours.

PEDIATRIC DOSAGE GUIDANCE:
• Bipolar: Start 2.5 mg SL BID, increase as needed up to 10 mg BID.
• For patch (approved for adults only): Start 3.8 mg/24 hours. May increase dosage to 5.7 mg/24 hours or 7.6 mg/24 hours after one week.
• Avoid food or drink for 10 minutes after taking. Do not swallow SL tablets; doing so will significantly reduce absorption and bioavailability.

MONITORING: Weight, waist circumference, glucose, lipids, BP, abnormal movements.

COST: SL: $$$: patch: $$$$$

SIDE EFFECTS:
• Most common: Akathisia (seems to be dose related), oral hypoesthesia (numbing of the tongue or decreased oral sensitivity), somnolence, fatigue, dizziness, increased appetite, EPS, weight gain. Application site reactions with patch.
• Serious but rare: Hypersensitivity reactions including anaphylaxis, angioedema, low blood pressure, rapid heart rate, swollen tongue, difficulty breathing, wheezing, or rash; orthostatic hypotension and syncope, particularly early in treatment.

MECHANISM, PHARMACOKINETICS, AND DRUG INTERACTIONS:
• Dopamine D2 and serotonin 5HT2A receptor antagonist.
• Metabolized by glucuronidation and CYP1A2; t ½: 24 hours. Inhibitor of 2D6; may double paroxetine levels. Smoking may induce metabolism and may lower levels of asenapine via 1A2 induction; adjust dosing. CYP1A2 inhibitors (eg, fluvoxamine) may increase levels of asenapine; adjust dose.
• Caution with antihypertensive agents and other drugs that can cause additive hypotension or bradycardia.

EVIDENCE AND CLINICAL PEARLS:
• Asenapine was studied in kids 12–17 with schizophrenia and was found to be no better than placebo.
• A three-week randomized study of 403 children (ages 10–17) with bipolar found significantly greater reduction in symptoms with asenapine compared to placebo.
• Has a receptor-binding profile similar to clozapine, although asenapine has very little anticholinergic activity.
• Weight gain does seem to be a problem in many adults, and rates are higher in pediatric patients.
• Pediatric patients more sensitive to dystonia during first few days of treatment with higher initial or faster escalation of dose.
• Contraindicated in patients with severe hepatic impairment due to seven-fold higher drug levels.
• Most useful for patients who don't like swallowing pills.

FUN FACT:
Black cherry flavor developed after patients complained about original tablets.

BREXPIPRAZOLE (Rexulti) Fact Sheet

BOTTOM LINE:
Brexpiprazole is a cousin of aripiprazole and is also a partial dopamine agonist. It has a very similar efficacy profile (including efficacy for depression in adults) and a similar side effect profile, but is much more expensive and has less data and experience in children. We recommend choosing the cheaper, generic aripiprazole.

PEDIATRIC FDA INDICATIONS:
Schizophrenia (13–17).

ADULT FDA INDICATIONS:
Schizophrenia; depression adjunct.

OFF-LABEL USES:
Dementia-related psychosis; borderline personality disorder.

DOSAGE FORMS:
Tablets: 0.25 mg, 0.5 mg, 1 mg, 2 mg, 3 mg, 4 mg.

DOSAGE GUIDANCE:
* Schizophrenia: Start 0.5 mg/day on days one through four, ↑ to 1 mg/day on days five through seven, then up to max 4 mg/day based on patient response. Usual dose 2–4 mg/day.
* Depression adjunct (indicated in adults only): Start 0.5 mg/day, ↑ at weekly intervals up to target 2 mg/day, max 3 mg/day.
* Dose timing: Like aripiprazole, can be taken in the morning or at night; may unpredictably cause drowsiness or insomnia.

MONITORING: Fasting glucose, lipids.

COST: $$$$$

SIDE EFFECTS:
* Most common: Weight gain, akathisia, somnolence.
* Serious but rare: Rare reports of reversible pathologic gambling and other impulse control problems (eating, spending, sexual).

MECHANISM, PHARMACOKINETICS, AND DRUG INTERACTIONS:
* Dopamine D2 and serotonin 5HT1A receptor partial agonist and serotonin 5HT2A receptor antagonist.
* Metabolized by CYP2D6 and CYP3A4; t ½: 91 hours.
* Use ½ usual dose in presence of 2D6 or 3A4 inhibitors or in known 2D6 poor metabolizers; ¼ dose if both 2D6 inhibitor/poor metabolizer and 3A4 inhibitor; double dose if also using 3A4 inducer.

CLINICAL PEARLS:
* As the name suggests, brexpiprazole is chemically and structurally related to its manufacturer's previous blockbuster aripiprazole (Abilify).
* Although the FDA-approved target dose for schizophrenia is 2–4 mg/day, 2 mg/day was no better than placebo in one of two preclinical registration studies.
* Unlike aripiprazole, brexpiprazole may not be effective in bipolar mania. It was no better than placebo at reducing symptoms in about 650 adult patients enrolled in two studies in acute mania. One study compared weight gain from brexpiprazole to aripiprazole and found a similar increase of about 5–10 pounds over a year.
* Once-a-day dosing with no regard to meals makes this an easy-to-use option.
* Generic/brand name mnemonic: "Brex is Rex" (thanks to Dr. Raj Mago).

FUN FACT:
Plan on seeing more trial results with Rexulti in the future, including those in patients with ADHD, PTSD, and agitation associated with Alzheimer's dementia.

CHLORPROMAZINE (Thorazine) Fact Sheet [G]

BOTTOM LINE:
Not commonly used in children, but may be considered in those with severe behavioral disturbances who may benefit from sedation.

PEDIATRIC FDA INDICATIONS:
Severe behavioral problems (6 months–17 years); **excessive motor activity and impulsivity.**

ADULT FDA INDICATIONS:
Psychosis; mania; nausea and vomiting; intractable hiccups.

OFF-LABEL USES:
Bipolar disorder; impulse control disorders.

DOSAGE FORMS:
- **Tablets (G):** 10 mg, 25 mg, 50 mg, 100 mg, 200 mg.
- **Oral concentrate (G):** 30 mg/mL, 100 mg/mL.
- **Injectable (G):** 25 mg/mL.

PEDIATRIC DOSAGE GUIDANCE:
Start 0.5 mg/kg Q4–6 hours PRN (eg, 20-kg or 45-lb child, use 10 mg Q4–6 hours PRN). In more severe patients, doses may range up to 50–100 mg/day or 200 mg/day in older children.

MONITORING: BP/P; ECG in patients at risk; prolactin in patients with symptoms, weight, waist circumference, lipids, glucose, abnormal movements.

COST: $$–$$$$ (depending on dose); oral concentrate: $$$$

SIDE EFFECTS:
- Most common: Sedation, orthostasis, tachycardia, drowsiness, dry mouth, constipation, blurred vision, prolactin elevation (sexual side effects, amenorrhea, galactorrhea), EPS, weight gain.
- Serious but rare: Skin pigmentation and ocular changes (both dose related); jaundice.

MECHANISM, PHARMACOKINETICS, AND DRUG INTERACTIONS:
- Dopamine D2 receptor antagonist.
- Metabolized primarily by CYP2D6, also 1A2 and 3A4. Patients who are poor metabolizers of CYP2D6 metabolize the drug more slowly; may have increased effects; t ½: 23–37 hours.
- CYP2D6 inhibitors (eg, fluoxetine, paroxetine, duloxetine, quinidine) may increase chlorpromazine levels.

EVIDENCE AND CLINICAL PEARLS:
- Although used in children (especially autistic and other neurodiverse kids and teens) for many years, data supporting its use are minimal and side effects may be significant.
- While chlorpromazine is approved for treating children with excessive motor activity and impulsivity (symptoms consistent with ADHD), stimulants were found to be more effective than antipsychotics in studies comparing the two.
- Chlorpromazine is a low-potency conventional (first-generation) antipsychotic; this leads to less EPS compared to high-potency agents (eg, haloperidol, fluphenazine) and to more anticholinergic side effects compared to mid- and high-potency agents (eg, perphenazine and haloperidol, respectively).
- Extremely sedating agent and often used for this effect. Dosing limited by orthostasis and sedation.

FUN FACT:
Thorazine was developed by a French surgeon in 1948 to induce relaxation and indifference in surgical patients.

Antipsychotics

CLOZAPINE (Clozaril, FazaClo, Versacloz) Fact Sheet [G]

BOTTOM LINE:
The only drug with convincing evidence based on years of clinical experience to help treatment-resistant schizophrenia, but only minimal data in children. Consider in severe cases, after failure of other agents.

PEDIATRIC FDA INDICATIONS:
None.

ADULT FDA INDICATIONS:
Treatment-resistant schizophrenia; reduction in risk of suicide in schizophrenia and schizoaffective disorder.

OFF-LABEL USES:
Treatment-resistant bipolar disorder; treatment-resistant aggression and violence.

DOSAGE FORMS:
- **Tablets (Clozaril):** 25 mg (scored), 100 mg (scored).
- **Tablets (G):** 25 mg (scored), 50 mg (scored), 100 mg (scored), 200 mg (scored).
- **Orally disintegrating tablets (FazaClo, [G]):** 12.5 mg, 25 mg, 100 mg, 150 mg, 200 mg.
- **Oral suspension (Versacloz):** 50 mg/mL.

PEDIATRIC DOSAGE GUIDANCE:
- No guidance on dosing in children and adolescents.
- Start 12.5 mg once or twice daily; ↑ gradually, in increments of 25–50 mg/day every few days to response. Max 900 mg/day (adolescents).
- If dosing is interrupted for ≥48 hours, must be re-titrated from 12.5–25 mg/day; may be increased more rapidly than initial titration, as tolerated.

MONITORING: Weight, waist circumference, glucose, lipids, BP/P; ECG in patients at risk, abnormal movements. Clinician must take a brief training course to enroll in REMS and then enroll patient. Before starting clozapine, ensure absolute neutrophil count (ANC) >1500; consult Clozapine REMS (https://www.newclozapinerems.com/home) for advice. Serum level monitoring can be useful in adults; minimal guidance for pediatric patients.

COST: $$$; ODT: $$$$; oral suspension: $$$$$

SIDE EFFECTS:
- Most common: Sedation, orthostatic hypotension, hypersalivation (place towel on pillow), weight gain (15–30 pound average weight gain after one year), constipation (risk of toxic megacolon if untreated), tachycardia (can treat with propranolol).
- Serious but rare: Potentially life-threatening agranulocytosis (1%–2%); periodic WBC testing (as above, see prescribing information for monitoring details) must occur. Recent concerns have arisen that clozapine carries a higher risk for hematologic neoplasms. While the relative risk is increased, the absolute risk remains low.

MECHANISM, PHARMACOKINETICS, AND DRUG INTERACTIONS:
- Dopamine D2 and serotonin 5HT2A receptor antagonist.
- Metabolized by several CYP450: 1A2, 2D6, and 3A4; t ½: 12 hours.
- Avoid use with drugs that may cause bone marrow suppression (eg, carbamazepine), lower seizure threshold, or have additive anticholinergic effects. Collapse, respiratory arrest, and cardiac arrest reported during initial clozapine treatment in patients taking benzodiazepines. Caution with P450 inhibitors and inducers. Smoking increases clozapine clearance by 30%–50%.

EVIDENCE AND CLINICAL PEARLS:
- Risk of neutropenia greatest within first six months, then incidence declines but can still occur.
- Divided doses may minimize some adverse effects (eg, hypotension, seizures).
- A growing number of adult case reports have been published linking very high clozapine serum levels to infection. Monitor levels and symptoms of toxicity closely, especially in patients hospitalized for infection.
- Limited data from three randomized clinical trials in children (as young as 6 years) showed better efficacy than haloperidol, olanzapine, and high-dose olanzapine.
- One small retrospective study in adolescents found decreased cannabis use and psychotic symptoms in those with concurrent psychosis and substance use.

FUN FACTS:
The Quiet Room is a compelling memoir written by patient Lori Schiller, who was an early user of clozapine.

HALOPERIDOL (Haldol) Fact Sheet [G]

BOTTOM LINE:
Haloperidol is an effective, inexpensive first-generation antipsychotic with a long history of experience and use even in kids, but clinical utility is limited due to potential for EPS, prolactin elevation, and TD.

PEDIATRIC FDA INDICATIONS:
Psychosis (3–17 years); **Tourette's disorder** (3–17 years); **severe behavioral problems** (3–17 years); **excessive motor activity, impulsivity** (3–17 years).

ADULT FDA INDICATIONS:
Psychosis; Tourette's disorder.

OFF-LABEL USES:
Bipolar disorder; impulse control disorders; delirium.

DOSAGE FORMS:
- **Tablets (G):** 0.5 mg (scored), 1 mg (scored), 2 mg (scored), 5 mg (scored), 10 mg (scored), 20 mg (scored).
- **Oral concentrate (G):** 2 mg/mL.
- **Injectable (G):** 5 mg/mL.
- **Long-acting injection (G):** 50 mg/mL and 100 mg/mL (see LAI fact sheet and table).

PEDIATRIC DOSAGE GUIDANCE:
- Weight-based guideline: 0.05–0.2 mg/kg/day.
- Start 0.25–0.5 mg/day; increase by 0.25–0.5 mg increments every five to seven days and adjust to lowest effective dose; usual range 0.5–5 mg/day, although doses up to 10 mg/day may be used in older children.

MONITORING: Prolactin, glucose, lipids, weight, waist circumference, EPS, abnormal movements.

COST: $

SIDE EFFECTS:
- Most common: EPS, headache, drowsiness, dry mouth, prolactin elevation (sexual side effects, amenorrhea, galactorrhea).
- Serious but rare: See class warnings in chapter introduction.

MECHANISM, PHARMACOKINETICS, AND DRUG INTERACTIONS:
- Dopamine D2 receptor antagonist.
- Metabolized primarily by CYP2D6, also 3A4; t ½: 21–24 hours. Patients who are poor metabolizers of CYP2D6 metabolize the drug more slowly; may have increased effects.
- CYP2D6 inhibitors (eg, fluoxetine, paroxetine, duloxetine, quinidine) may increase haloperidol levels. May inhibit CYP2D6; caution with substrates of 2D6 as haloperidol may increase their levels and effects.

EVIDENCE AND CLINICAL PEARLS:
- Older data in children with Tourette's, severe behavioral disorders, and psychosis show some benefit. Haloperidol is also the most well-studied first-generation antipsychotic in treating autistic children.
- Although haloperidol is approved for treating children with excessive motor activity and impulsivity (symptoms consistent with ADHD), stimulants have been shown to be more effective than antipsychotics in studies comparing the two.
- Haloperidol is a high-potency conventional (first-generation) antipsychotic; this leads to more EPS compared to mid- or low-potency agents (eg, perphenazine or chlorpromazine, respectively) and to less sedation, less orthostasis, and fewer anticholinergic side effects compared to low-potency agents (eg, chlorpromazine).
- Relatively lower seizure side effect risk compared to lower-potency agents.
- Availability of short-acting injectable and oral liquid formulations allows for more flexibility in administration.
- Long-acting injectable decanoate formulation allows option for patients who don't take oral formation reliably.

FUN FACT:
Haldol was discovered in 1958 by Paul Janssen, the founder of Belgian pharmaceutical company Janssen Pharmaceutica.

Antipsychotics

LURASIDONE (Latuda) Fact Sheet

BOTTOM LINE:
This drug offers some advantages, including no need for titration, once-daily dosing, relatively low-moderate metabolic profile, and relatively low QT prolongation risk. However, its use is limited by the need to administer with ≥350 calories of food, potential for drug interactions, and side effects including sedation, akathisia, and EPS, not to mention relatively minimal data (and certainly no long-term data) in kids.

PEDIATRIC FDA INDICATIONS:
Schizophrenia (13–17 years); **bipolar I depression** (as monotherapy and adjunct, 10–17 years).

ADULT FDA INDICATIONS:
Schizophrenia; bipolar I depression (as monotherapy and adjunct).

OFF-LABEL USES:
Mixed depression; treatment-resistant depression; impulse control disorders.

DOSAGE FORMS:
Tablets: 20 mg, 40 mg, 60 mg, 80 mg, 120 mg.

PEDIATRIC DOSAGE GUIDANCE:
Start 40 mg QD, with food (at least 350 calories); no titration required. Usual dose 40–80 mg/day. Max dose 80 mg/day for adolescents vs 160 mg/day in adults.

MONITORING: Weight, waist circumference, glucose, lipids, BP/P, abnormal movements.

COST: $$$$$

SIDE EFFECTS:
- Most common: Somnolence (dose related), EPS, akathisia (dose related), nausea and vomiting, weight gain.
- Serious but rare: Orthostatic hypotension and syncope reported (rarely).

MECHANISM, PHARMACOKINETICS, AND DRUG INTERACTIONS:
- Dopamine D2 and serotonin 5HT2A and 5HT7 antagonist; serotonin 5HT1A partial agonist.
- Metabolized primarily through CYP3A4; t ½: 18 hours.
- Avoid use with medications that cause orthostasis, potent 3A4 inhibitors (eg, ketoconazole, clarithromycin), or inducers (eg, rifampin, St. John's wort, carbamazepine). Exercise caution/monitor when using in combination with moderate 3A4 inhibitors (eg, diltiazem); decrease lurasidone dose by 50% in patients taking moderate 3A4 inhibitors.

EVIDENCE AND CLINICAL PEARLS:
- Newest indication of bipolar depression in kids is based on a six-week randomized double-blind placebo-controlled study of 347 kids receiving lurasidone 20–80 mg/day or placebo. Lurasidone-treated patients had a statistically significant larger improvement in symptoms of bipolar depression, with an effect size of 0.45 (as measured by Children's Depression Rating Scale, Revised).
- A placebo-controlled study of lurasidone in irritability associated with autism found it no better than placebo, and 13 out of 18 kids ages 6–12 years experienced vomiting.
- While using lurasidone in bipolar depression has not been associated with an increase in the development of mania, its efficacy in treating manic episodes has not been established, so its use should be reserved for depressive episodes.
- Administration with food (at least 350 calories) increases bioavailability two-fold and peak serum levels roughly three-fold; fat content of meal is not important.
- Appears to be relatively weight-neutral and to have little effect on cardiometabolic parameters in company-sponsored trials, although post-marketing observations have been limited, particularly in kids.

FUN FACT:
One unique feature of Latuda is its high affinity for the 5HT7 receptor, which has been linked to depression, learning/memory, cognition, anxiety, and pain. Unfortunately, to date, Latuda has shown no clear benefit over other second-generation antipsychotics on these measures.

OLANZAPINE (Lybalvi, Symbyax, Zyprexa) Fact Sheet [G]

BOTTOM LINE:
Its high risk for weight gain and metabolic complications make it a second-line choice for kids and adolescents. Consider co-administering metformin to prevent weight gain.

PEDIATRIC FDA INDICATIONS:
Schizophrenia (13–17 years); **bipolar acute mania** (13–17 years); **bipolar I depression** (with fluoxetine, as Symbyax, 10–17 years).

ADULT FDA INDICATIONS:
Schizophrenia; acute or mixed bipolar I manic episodes, as monotherapy or adjunct; maintenance treatment of bipolar disorder; bipolar I depression (with fluoxetine, as Symbyax); treatment-resistant unipolar depression (with fluoxetine); acute agitation in schizophrenia and bipolar mania (injectable form).

OFF-LABEL USES:
Behavioral disturbances; impulse control disorders.

DOSAGE FORMS:
* **Tablets (G):** 2.5 mg, 5 mg, 7.5 mg, 10 mg, 15 mg, 20 mg.
* **Orally disintegrating tablets (Zyprexa Zydis, [G]):** 5 mg, 10 mg, 15 mg, 20 mg.
* **IM injection (G):** 10 mg.
* **Long-acting injection (Zyprexa Relprevv):** 210 mg, 300 mg, 405 mg (see LAI fact sheet and table).
* **Fixed-combination capsules with fluoxetine (Symbyax, [G]):** 3/25 mg, 6/25 mg, 12/25 mg, 6/50 mg, 12/50 mg olanzapine/fluoxetine.
* **Fixed-combination tablets with samidorphan (Lybalvi):** 5/10 mg, 10/10 mg, 15/10 mg, 20/10 mg olanzapine/samidorphan.

PEDIATRIC DOSAGE GUIDANCE:
* Schizophrenia and acute mania: Start most at 2.5–5 mg QD; may ↑ by 5 mg QD, in weekly increments, to target dose 10 mg QD; max 20 mg QD.
* Bipolar depression (Symbyax, fixed combination with fluoxetine): Start 3/25 mg QPM, ↑ as indicated to target dose 6/25 mg olanzapine/fluoxetine; max dose 12/50 mg.
* For Lybalvi, dose as above using equivalent olanzapine component. Do not divide or combine Lybalvi strengths.

MONITORING: Weight, waist circumference, glucose, lipids, prolactin if symptoms, abnormal movements.

COST: $; combination with fluoxetine: $$; Lybalvi: $$$$$

SIDE EFFECTS:
* Most common: Somnolence (dose related), dry mouth (dose related), constipation, weight gain (up to 40% incidence and may be substantial; 10–30 pounds weight gain is common), increased appetite, EPS (dose related); increased LFTs; increased prolactin.
* Serious but rare: Rare but potentially fatal drug reaction with eosinophilia and systemic symptoms (DRESS) possible; often starting as rash that may spread, fever, swollen lymph nodes, and elevated eosinophils.

MECHANISM, PHARMACOKINETICS, AND DRUG INTERACTIONS:
* Dopamine D2 and serotonin 5HT2A receptor antagonist.
* Metabolized by CYP1A2, 2D6 (minor), and direct glucuronidation; t ½: 1–2 days.
* CYP1A2 inducers (eg, carbamazepine, ritonavir, smoking) may reduce olanzapine levels by 50%; CYP1A2 inhibitors (eg, fluvoxamine) may increase olanzapine bioavailability by 50%–100%. Adjust olanzapine dosing in presence of 1A2 inducers or inhibitors.

EVIDENCE AND CLINICAL PEARLS:
* Compared to adults, children and adolescents are more likely to gain more weight, experience greater sedation, and have greater increases in LDL cholesterol, total cholesterol, triglycerides, prolactin, and liver transaminase levels.
* Newly approved combination with opioid antagonist samidorphan reduces risk of weight gain, but moderate weight gain risk nevertheless. Avoid use of opioids.

FUN FACT:
Olanzapine has been studied and is used for chemotherapy-induced nausea and vomiting.

Antipsychotics

PALIPERIDONE (Invega) Fact Sheet [G]

BOTTOM LINE:
Invega looks like risperidone without drug-drug interactions, but with more QT interval prolongation, more tachycardia, possibly more EPS, and the same amount of hyperprolactinemia. These significant disadvantages, and relatively fewer data in kids, make it a second-line option.

PEDIATRIC FDA INDICATIONS:
Schizophrenia (12–17 years).

ADULT FDA INDICATIONS:
Schizophrenia; schizoaffective disorder.

OFF-LABEL USES:
Bipolar disorder; behavioral disturbances; impulse control disorders.

DOSAGE FORMS:
- **Controlled-release tablets (G):** 1.5 mg, 3 mg, 6 mg, 9 mg (not breakable).
- **Monthly long-acting injection (Invega Sustenna):** 39 mg, 78 mg, 117 mg, 156 mg, 234 mg (see LAI fact sheet and table).
- **Every-3-month long-acting injection (Invega Trinza):** 273 mg, 410 mg, 546 mg, 819 mg (see LAI fact sheet and table).
- **Every-6-month long-acting injection (Invega Hafyera):** 1,092 mg/3.5 mL, 1,560 mg/5 mL (see LAI fact sheet and table).

PEDIATRIC DOSAGE GUIDANCE:
- Start 3 mg QAM, which may be the effective dose; if required, may ↑ by 3 mg/day at intervals of >5 days to max 6 mg/day (weight <51 kg) or 12 mg/day (weight ≥51 kg). Dose adjustment in renal impairment.
- Paliperidone 3 mg, 6 mg, 9 mg, and 12 mg roughly equivalent to 1–2 mg, 2–4 mg, 4–6 mg, and 6–8 mg risperidone, respectively.

MONITORING: Weight, waist circumference, glucose, lipids, prolactin, abnormal movements.

COST: $$$

SIDE EFFECTS:
- Most common: Akathisia, EPS (dose related), tremor, tachycardia, somnolence (especially adolescents), weight gain, prolactin elevation.
- Serious but rare: Modest increase in QT. Orthostatic hypotension and syncope reported. Rarely, controlled-release tablet may cause GI obstruction in patients with strictures (either pathologic or iatrogenic). Esophageal dysmotility and aspiration possible; use caution in patients at risk for aspiration pneumonia (eg, those with developmental disorders).

MECHANISM, PHARMACOKINETICS, AND DRUG INTERACTIONS:
- Dopamine D2 and serotonin 5HT2A receptor antagonist.
- Not metabolized by liver; t ½: 23 hours.
- Avoid use with drugs known to prolong the QT interval or to cause orthostasis. Paliperidone is the principal active metabolite of risperidone; therefore, avoid use with risperidone. Minimal drug interactions.

EVIDENCE AND CLINICAL PEARLS:
- An eight-week double-blind randomized trial in 228 adolescents with schizophrenia, with a maintenance period of 18 weeks, found paliperidone was equally effective as aripiprazole.
- An eight-week observational study in 15 kids with mania reported remission in 47% of patients treated with paliperidone.
- An open-label study in autistic kids suggested efficacy.
- Warn your patients that they may find capsules in their stool. These are empty "ghost pills." Invega (and Concerta; see fact sheet) is an extended-release tablet based on the OROS osmotic delivery system, which releases medication from a hard shell.
- Swallow whole, with fluids; do not chew, divide, or crush.
- In adult studies, paliperidone is not effective in acute mania even with lithium or valproate.
- Along with risperidone, causes the most EPS and hyperprolactinemia of all the second-generation antipsychotics.

FUN FACT:
First drug with FDA approval for schizoaffective disorder in adults, allowing Janssen to carve out a new marketing niche and separate this drug from its competitors (at least from a commercial perspective).

PERPHENAZINE (Trilafon) Fact Sheet [G]

BOTTOM LINE:
Well-tolerated and inexpensive alternative to second-generation antipsychotics, especially when trying to avoid EPS and metabolic side effects; however, efficacy data in kids are more limited compared to newer agents.

PEDIATRIC FDA INDICATIONS:
Schizophrenia (12+ years).

ADULT FDA INDICATIONS:
Schizophrenia; severe nausea and vomiting.

OFF-LABEL USES:
Bipolar disorder; behavioral disturbances; impulse control disorders.

DOSAGE FORMS:
Tablets (G): 2 mg, 4 mg, 8 mg, 16 mg.

PEDIATRIC DOSAGE GUIDANCE:
Ages >12: Start 4 mg BID; adjust to lowest effective dose. Dose range 8–16 mg BID–QID; max FDA-approved dose for non-hospitalized patients is 24 mg/day, but hospitalized psychotic patients may be dosed up to 64 mg/day (adults).

MONITORING: Prolactin, lipids, glucose, EPS, abnormal movements.

COST: $

SIDE EFFECTS:
- Most common: EPS, headache, drowsiness, dry mouth, prolactin elevation (sexual side effects, amenorrhea, galactorrhea).
- Serious but rare: Tachycardia (especially with sudden marked increase in dose).

MECHANISM, PHARMACOKINETICS, AND DRUG INTERACTIONS:
- Dopamine D2 receptor antagonist.
- Metabolized primarily by CYP2D6; t ½: 9–12 hours. May inhibit CYP2D6. Poor metabolizers of CYP2D6 metabolize the drug more slowly; may have increased effects.
- CYP2D6 inhibitors (eg, fluoxetine, paroxetine, duloxetine, quinidine) may increase perphenazine levels. Caution with substrates of 2D6 as perphenazine may increase their levels and effects.

EVIDENCE AND CLINICAL PEARLS:
- No clinical trial data in children or adolescents with schizophrenia, but FDA indicated and used in kids by some clinicians based on experience as well as results from efficacy studies in adults.
- Based on an 18-month randomized trial of 1,493 adult patients with schizophrenia (CATIE trial), perphenazine appears similar in efficacy and EPS compared to second-generation antipsychotics (olanzapine, quetiapine, risperidone, ziprasidone).
- Perphenazine is an intermediate-potency conventional (first-generation) antipsychotic; this leads to less EPS compared to high-potency agents (eg, haloperidol, fluphenazine) and to less sedation, less orthostasis, and fewer anticholinergic side effects compared to low-potency agents (eg, chlorpromazine).
- Fewer metabolic effects (weight gain, glucose, lipids) than some antipsychotics.

FUN FACT:
Perphenazine has long been available in a formulation with amitriptyline (a tricyclic antidepressant) called Triavil. This combination antipsychotic/antidepressant was first available in 1965, foreshadowing the next such combination drug (Symbyax) by 38 years.

Antipsychotics

QUETIAPINE (Seroquel) Fact Sheet [G]

BOTTOM LINE:
Lower risk for EPS and a broad spectrum of efficacy make this an appealing first-choice agent. However, sedation, weight gain, and orthostasis may limit use. Dosing at bedtime, or switching to XR, may help reduce daytime sedation.

PEDIATRIC FDA INDICATIONS:
Schizophrenia (13–17 years); **bipolar mania** (10–17 years).

ADULT FDA INDICATIONS:
Schizophrenia; bipolar, manic/mixed; bipolar I or II depression; maintenance treatment for bipolar; major depression, as adjunct.

OFF-LABEL USES:
Insomnia; anxiety disorders; behavioral disturbances; impulse control disorders.

DOSAGE FORMS:
- **Tablets (G):** 25 mg, 50 mg, 100 mg, 200 mg, 300 mg, 400 mg.
- **ER tablets (G):** 50 mg, 150 mg, 200 mg, 300 mg, 400 mg.

PEDIATRIC DOSAGE GUIDANCE:
- Adolescents: Start 25 mg BID or 50 mg XR QHS, ↑ dose by 50–100 mg/day increments every one to four days to target/max dose 400–600 mg/day (mania) or 400–800 mg/day (schizophrenia).
- Max dose for <9 years: 400 mg/day.

MONITORING: Prolactin if symptoms, lipids, glucose, BP, weight, waist circumference, abnormal movements.

COST: $

SIDE EFFECTS:
- Most common: Somnolence, hypotension, dry mouth, dizziness, weight gain, increased appetite, fatigue, nausea, vomiting, tachycardia, EPS, abnormal movements.
- Serious but rare: Increases in BP occurred in pediatric studies vs orthostasis in adults (15% had systolic elevation >20 mmHg and 40% had diastolic elevation >10 mmHg).

MECHANISM, PHARMACOKINETICS, AND DRUG INTERACTIONS:
- Dopamine D2 and serotonin 5HT2A receptor antagonist.
- Metabolized by CYP3A4; t ½: 6 hours (ER: 7 hours).
- Avoid or use caution with agents that may cause additional orthostasis. CYP3A4 inducers (eg, carbamazepine) may lower quetiapine levels; CYP3A4 inhibitors (eg, erythromycin, ketoconazole) may increase quetiapine levels. Adjust quetiapine dose in presence of CYP3A4 inducers or inhibitors.

EVIDENCE AND CLINICAL PEARLS:
- A six-week randomized controlled trial in 220 adolescents with schizophrenia found quetiapine was significantly more effective than placebo at reducing psychotic symptoms.
- A three-week randomized trial in 277 kids (ages 10–17) with bipolar disorder found significantly higher remission rates with quetiapine compared to placebo.
- A four-week randomized trial in 50 kids (ages 12–18) with bipolar disorder found significantly higher remission rates with quetiapine than divalproex.
- A study in bipolar depression in kids (ages 10–17) did not find quetiapine XR more effective than placebo. Two open-label studies in autism did not find it to be effective either.
- Swallow XR tablet whole; do not break, crush, or chew; switch between IR and XR at the same total daily dose; dose adjustments may be necessary based on response and tolerability.
- If patient discontinues drug >1 week, retitrate dose as with initial therapy.
- Quetiapine abuse has been reported, particularly in incarcerated adult populations.
- Nearly 20% of children gained >7% of body weight (adjusted for usual growth) after 26 weeks of quetiapine.

FUN FACT:
Cataracts developed in initial studies with beagle dogs; human studies have not shown an association. However, the label still recommends a slit-lamp exam every six months.

RISPERIDONE (Risperdal) Fact Sheet [G]

BOTTOM LINE:
Risperidone offers more efficacy and safety data in kids than other antipsychotics and is often used first-line in autistic kids, but you need to expect and monitor for EPS, prolactinemia, and weight gain. Consider co-administration with benztropine to prevent EPS and/or metformin to prevent weight gain.

PEDIATRIC FDA INDICATIONS:
Schizophrenia (13–17 years); **bipolar mania, monotherapy and adjunctive** (10–17 years); **irritability in autism** (5–17 years).

ADULT FDA INDICATIONS:
Schizophrenia; bipolar disorder, manic/mixed.

OFF-LABEL USES:
Bipolar depression; behavioral disturbances; impulse control disorders; Tourette's disorder.

DOSAGE FORMS:
- **Tablets (G):** 0.25 mg, 0.5 mg, 1 mg, 2 mg, 3 mg, 4 mg.
- **Oral solution (G):** 1 mg/mL.
- **Orally disintegrating tablets (Risperdal M-Tab, [G]):** 0.25 mg, 0.5 mg, 1 mg, 2 mg, 3 mg, 4 mg.
- **Long-acting injection (Risperdal Consta):** 12.5 mg, 25 mg, 37.5 mg, 50 mg (see LAI fact sheet and table).
- **Long-acting injection (Perseris):** 90 mg, 120 mg (see LAI fact sheet and table).

PEDIATRIC DOSAGE GUIDANCE:
- Autism (children ≥5 years): If <15 kg (33 lbs), use with caution. For 15–20 kg (33–44 lbs), start 0.25 mg/day, ↑ to 0.5 mg/day after ≥4 days. If response insufficient, may ↑ by 0.25 mg/day in ≥2-week intervals; give QD or BID. For ≥20 kg (44 lbs), start 0.5 mg/day; may ↑ to 1 mg/day after ≥4 days. If response insufficient, may ↑ dose by 0.5 mg/day in ≥2-week intervals; give QD or BID.
- Bipolar mania or schizophrenia (children): Start 0.5 mg QD; ↑ in increments of 0.5–1 mg/day at intervals ≥24 hours to target dose of 2–3 mg/day; doses >3 mg/day do not confer additional benefit and are associated with increased side effects.

MONITORING: Weight, waist circumference, glucose, lipids, BP; prolactin, abnormal movements.

COST: $

SIDE EFFECTS:
- Most common: EPS, somnolence, anxiety, dizziness, salivary hypersecretion, fatigue, prolactin elevation, weight gain, increased appetite.
- Serious but rare: Orthostatic hypotension may occur, particularly at higher doses or with rapid titration. Hyperprolactinemia with clinical symptoms (sexual side effects, galactorrhea, amenorrhea).

MECHANISM, PHARMACOKINETICS, AND DRUG INTERACTIONS:
- Dopamine D2 and serotonin 5HT2A receptor antagonist.
- Metabolized by CYP2D6; t ½: 20 hours.
- CYP2D6 inhibitors (eg, fluoxetine, paroxetine, duloxetine, quinidine) may increase effects of risperidone; reduce risperidone dose. Carbamazepine reduces levels and effects of risperidone; may need to double risperidone dose.

EVIDENCE AND CLINICAL PEARLS:
- Seven published trials have reported efficacy of risperidone in adolescents with schizophrenia (two open label, two comparisons with olanzapine and haloperidol, two comparisons with olanzapine, and one randomized placebo-controlled study).
- A three-week randomized trial in 169 children (ages 10–17) with bipolar mania found significantly higher remission rates with risperidone compared to placebo. A six-week randomized trial in 66 kids (ages 8–18) with bipolar mania found significantly higher remission rates with risperidone compared to divalproex. An eight-week open-label trial in 279 kids (ages 6–15) with bipolar mania found higher response rates with risperidone compared to both lithium and divalproex sodium; responses to lithium vs divalproex were similar.
- In autistic kids, associated irritability as well as symptoms of aggression toward others, deliberate self-injuriousness, temper tantrums, and quickly changing moods are improved.
- In studies with kids, about ⅓ gained more than 7% of body weight, and over 80% had elevations in prolactin (dose related, more frequent in girls than boys).
- Along with paliperidone, causes the most EPS and hyperprolactinemia of all the second-generation antipsychotics.
- When reinitiating after discontinuation, initial titration schedule should be followed.

FUN FACT:
Risperdal M-tabs are marketed in other countries as Risperdal Quicklets.

Antipsychotics

ZIPRASIDONE (Geodon) Fact Sheet [G]

BOTTOM LINE:
Growing body of research supports both efficacy and safety in kids. However, the disadvantages—including twice-daily dosing, need to administer with food, and relatively great QT prolongation—give us some pause in our pediatric patients.

PEDIATRIC FDA INDICATIONS:
None.

ADULT FDA INDICATIONS:
Schizophrenia; bipolar disorder, acute treatment of manic/mixed episode; maintenance treatment of bipolar disorder, as adjunct; acute agitation in patients with schizophrenia (IM only).

OFF-LABEL USES:
Bipolar disorder; behavioral disturbances; impulse control disorders; Tourette's disorder.

DOSAGE FORMS:
• **Capsules (G):** 20 mg, 40 mg, 60 mg, 80 mg.
• **Injection (G):** 20 mg/mL.

PEDIATRIC DOSAGE GUIDANCE:
• No guidance on dosing in children and adolescents.
• Schizophrenia, bipolar disorder: Start 20 mg BID (40 mg BID for acute mania) with meals for two to three days; ↑ by 40 mg/day increments; can usually ↑ rather quickly to target dose 60–80 mg BID. Max approved dose is 160 mg/day, though can go higher in some patients; there are some safety data for doses up to 320 mg/day.
• Schizophrenia, acute agitation (IM injection): 10 mg Q2 hours or 20 mg Q4 hours; max 40 mg/day. Replace with oral therapy as soon as possible.

MONITORING: Weight, waist circumference, glucose, lipids; ECG, abnormal movements.

COST: $

SIDE EFFECTS:
• Most common: Somnolence, dizziness, akathisia, rash (5%), weight gain, EPS, abnormal movements.
• Serious but rare: May result in minor QTc prolongation (dose related; 10 msec at 160 mg/day). Clinically relevant prolongation (>500 msec) rare (0.06%) and less than placebo (0.23%). Significant QTc prolongation has been associated with the development of malignant ventricular arrhythmias (torsades de pointes) and sudden death. Avoid in patients receiving other drugs that prolong QTc, or who have hypokalemia, hypomagnesemia, bradycardia, or persistent QTc > 500 msec. Patients with symptoms of dizziness, palpitations, or syncope should receive further cardiac evaluation. Drug reaction with eosinophilia and systemic symptoms (DRESS) has been reported with ziprasidone exposure. DRESS begins as a rash that can spread all over the body; it may include swollen lymph nodes, fever, and damage to organs such as the heart, liver, pancreas, or kidneys, and is sometimes fatal. Discontinue ziprasidone if DRESS is suspected.

MECHANISM, PHARMACOKINETICS, AND DRUG INTERACTIONS:
• Dopamine D2 and serotonin 5HT2A receptor antagonist.
• Metabolized in liver principally by aldehyde oxidase; less than ⅓ of clearance mediated by CYP450: CYP3A4 (major), and CYP1A2 (minor); t ½: 7 hours.
• Avoid use with other drugs that prolong QT interval.

EVIDENCE AND CLINICAL PEARLS:
• One six-week (with 26-week open-label extension) placebo-controlled randomized trial in adolescents with schizophrenia failed to show separation between ziprasidone and placebo in efficacy measures.
• A four-week randomized trial in 237 children and adolescents (ages 10–17) found significantly greater symptom reduction and response rates with ziprasidone compared to placebo.
• Only limited data with ziprasidone in autistic kids or kids with Tourette's.
• Administer twice daily, ideally with meals; ingestion of several hundred calories is necessary to increase absorption up to two-fold.
• Causes less weight gain than clozapine, olanzapine, quetiapine, or risperidone.
• Average increase in QTc greater than any other second-generation antipsychotics, although not much more than for quetiapine. Post-marketing surveillance has shown one or two instances of torsades de pointes possibly related to ziprasidone use.

FUN FACT:
The brand name Geodon has been suggested to bring to mind the phrase "down (don) to earth (geo)," referring to the goals of the medication.

LONG-ACTING INJECTABLE (LAI) Antipsychotics

INTRODUCTION: IS THERE A ROLE FOR LAIS IN CHILDREN AND ADOLESCENTS?

LAIs are sometimes used for children and adolescents who need antipsychotics for severe illness but have difficulty consistently taking oral meds. A 2017 literature review found a few case series and case reports on such children, including a total of 36 individuals with a mean age of about 12. Most were boys, the most common diagnosis was bipolar disorder, and the majority of patients were on either risperidone or paliperidone palmitate. Most of these kids improved on the LAI, and weight gain was the most common side effect (www.tinyurl.com/yb4wq5zb).

Much more research is available for adults, and while results are mixed, in naturalistic studies that focus on real-world patients who are most likely to be prescribed LAIs (that is, those who have a history of non-adherence), it's clear that switching to injectables decreases the risk of hospitalization (Kishimoto T et al, *J Clin Psychiatry* 2013;74(10):957–965).

DECIDING AMONG THE LAIS

General Notes on LAIs

- It's best to choose an LAI version of an oral medication that your patient has already taken, so that you can be more confident that the agent is effective and tolerable.
- Be patient; full therapeutic effects of LAIs take longer than orals—ie, several months. Don't adjust the dose prematurely.
- Consider oral overlap. Agents differ on how quickly you can titrate up the dose. This is important because patients requiring gradual titration will need oral pills to make sure they have a decent serum level right away. This process is called the "oral overlap," and it has two disadvantages. First, it makes the process of dosing a bit more complex (not a huge deal); second, if the patient is refusing to take oral meds (but accepting an injection, either under court order or voluntarily), you'll have to choose a different LAI or risk a decompensation while waiting for levels to become therapeutic.
- *Never* initiate an LAI on a patient who has a history of neuroleptic malignant syndrome on any antipsychotic. That's just asking for trouble.

LAI Options

There's a pretty comprehensive table on the following pages that reports, for each LAI, the **FDA indication(s), medication names, costs, available strengths, dosing information,** and **pharmacokinetics** (need for oral overlap and dosing interval). But first, we'll give you a shorthand version of the most relevant **clinical pearls** below:

First-generation antipsychotics

- **Fluphenazine (Prolixin Decanoate)**—Dosed every two to three weeks. Injections are painful. Cheap, but relatively high risk of EPS and TD. Oral overlap required.
- **Haloperidol (Haldol Decanoate)**—Dosed monthly. As cheap as Prolixin, and since it's dosed less often and the pharmacokinetics are more predictable, it's generally the better choice among first-generation antipsychotics. Oral overlap required, although some use a "loading dose" method (20 times oral dose, followed by 10–15 times oral dose in subsequent months) that requires no oral overlap.

Second-generation antipsychotics

- **Aripiprazole (Abilify Maintena)**—Dosed monthly. Comes in two strengths (300 and 400 mg). Oral overlap required for 14 days. Deltoid or gluteal injection. Expensive. Good side effect profile.
- **Aripiprazole lauroxil (Aristada)**—Dosed monthly, every six weeks, or every two months. Smallest dose (441 mg monthly) may be given deltoid or gluteal; other doses must be given gluteal. Dosing interval flexibility makes this formulation appealing, although oral overlap is required for 21 days. You can forgo the oral overlap if you give your patient a dose of **Aristada Initio** 675 mg plus 30 mg oral aripiprazole on the same day as your first dose of Aristada. First dose of Aristada may be delayed up to 10 days after Initio. Expensive. Good side effect profile.
- **Olanzapine (Zyprexa Relprevv)**—Dosed either every two weeks or monthly, depending on the dose needed. May be the worst LAI choice for multiple reasons. High potential for weight gain. There's a small risk of a post-injection delirium/sedation syndrome, occurring in less than 1% of patients, caused by accidental intravascular injection. For this reason, you have to give the injection at a registered health care facility where patients can be continuously monitored for at least three hours after the injection. Restricted use requires physician and facility registration, and additional paperwork with Eli Lilly's program. High cost, restriction of use, monitoring requirement, and risk of adverse outcome all limit use severely. Gluteal injection only. Expensive. No oral overlap.
- **Paliperidone palmitate monthly (Invega Sustenna)**—Monthly dosing. Less painful injection than Risperdal Consta or Zyprexa Relprevv. No oral overlap required; need for two separate loading injections makes initiation a bit more complicated. First two doses deltoid; subsequent doses may be deltoid or gluteal. Expensive. No oral overlap and potential to transition to every-three-month and every-six-month formulations are appealing features.
- **Paliperidone palmitate every three months (Invega Trinza)**—Every-three-month dosing, but your patient must have done well on monthly injections of Sustenna for at least four months before switching to Trinza. Deltoid or gluteal injection. Must shake syringe vigorously for at least 15 seconds to ensure uniform suspension of long-acting particles and prevent clogging in needle. Expensive. No oral overlap.

Antipsychotics

- **Paliperidone palmitate every six months (Invega Hafyera)**—Every-six-month dosing, but your patient must have done well on monthly injections of Sustenna for at least four months or on Trinza for at least one three-month cycle. Gluteal injection. Switching from lower doses of Sustenna (39, 78, 117 mg) or Trinza (273, 410 mg) was not studied, so not recommended. Must shake syringe vigorously for at least 30 seconds to ensure uniform suspension and prevent clogging in needle. Expensive.
- **Risperidone (Risperdal Consta)**—Every-two-week dosing; three-week oral overlap. Cumbersome; must be refrigerated and shaken for at least 10 seconds. Painful deltoid or gluteal injection. Expensive.
- **Risperidone (Perseris)**—Monthly dosing option for risperidone, an improvement over the every-two-week dosing of Consta. No oral overlap. It's the first LAI to be dosed subcutaneously (into the abdomen) rather than a deep and more painful IM injection. Note that the highest dose of Perseris is equivalent to 4 mg/day of oral risperidone, so this isn't a good option for patients on higher doses. Expensive.

TABLE 8: Long-Acting Injectable Antipsychotics

Generic Name (Brand Name) Year FDA Approved [G] denotes generic availability	Relevant FDA Indication(s)	Available Strengths	Oral Overlap	Dosing Interval	Initial Dosing	Maintenance Dose	Cost for Monthly Supply at Average Dose (August 2022)
First-Generation Antipsychotics							
Fluphenazine decanoate [G] (Prolixin Decanoate¹) 1972	Schizophrenia	25 mg/mL	Continue total oral dose for 2–3 days, then ↓ by 50% increments every 2–3 days until discontinued (by next injection)	2–3 weeks	1.25x total daily oral dose Q2–3 weeks (5–11 yrs: 3.125–12.5 mg; ≥12 yrs: 6.25–25 mg)	Increase in increments of 3.125–12.5 mg; do not exceed 25 mg per dose	$ [G]
Haloperidol decanoate [G] (Haldol Decanoate) 1986	Schizophrenia	50, 100 mg/mL	Decrease oral dose by 50% after first injection, then discontinue after second injections (third for some patients); alternatively, no oral overlap if loading dose of 20x oral given	4 weeks	10–15x total oral daily dose Q4 weeks. First dose should be ≤100 mg; if higher dose needed, give remainder in 1–2 weeks. Alternatively, 20x total oral daily dose if loading dose with no oral overlap.	10–15x total oral daily dose Q4 weeks with either method	$ [G] $$$$ Haldol Dec
Second-Generation Antipsychotics							
Aripiprazole (Abilify Maintena) 2013	Schizophrenia Bipolar disorder	300, 400 mg vials and prefilled syringes	For 14 days	4 weeks	400 mg Q4 weeks	400 mg Q4 weeks; decrease to 300 mg Q4 weeks if side effects (estimated equivalence is 20 mg/day oral ~ 300 mg IM monthly and 30 mg/day oral ~ 400 mg IM monthly)	$$$$$
Aripiprazole lauroxil (Aristada) 2015	Schizophrenia	441, 662, 882, 1064 mg	For 21 days	Monthly, every 6 weeks, or every 2 months	441, 662, or 882 mg monthly (equivalent to 10, 15, and 20 mg/day); or 882 mg every 6 weeks (15 mg/day); or 1064 mg every 2 months (15 mg/day)	Continue initial dosing or adjust based on clinical response	$$$$$
Aripiprazole lauroxil (Aristada Initio) 2018	Schizophrenia	675 mg syringes	Aripiprazole 30 mg PO x1 dose	See Aristada above	To be given as single initial dose, in conjunction with Aristada as above (on same day or within 10 days of Initio)	See above	$$$$$
Olanzapine (Zyprexa Relprevv) 2009	Schizophrenia	210, 300, 405 mg vials	No overlap	2–4 weeks	10 mg/day oral: 210 mg Q2 weeks x4 doses or 405 mg Q4 weeks x2 doses; 15 mg/day oral: 300 mg Q2 weeks x4 doses; 20 mg/day oral: 300 mg Q2 weeks	10 mg/day oral: 150 mg Q2 weeks or 300 mg Q4 weeks; 15 mg/day oral: 210 mg Q2 weeks or 405 mg Q4 weeks; 20 mg/day oral: 300 mg Q2 weeks; Maximum dose: 300 mg Q2 weeks or 405 mg Q4 weeks	$$$$$

Generic Name (Brand Name) Year FDA Approved [G] denotes generic availability	Relevant FDA Indication(s)	Available Strengths	Oral Overlap	Dosing Interval	Initial Dosing	Maintenance Dose	Cost for Monthly Supply at Average Dose (August 2022)
Paliperidone palmitate (Invega Sustenna) 2009	Schizophrenia Schizoaffective disorder (monotherapy or adjunct)	39, 78, 117, 156, 234 mg prefilled syringes	No overlap	4 weeks	234 mg IM in deltoid, then 156 mg 1 week later	117 mg 3 weeks after 2nd dose then Q month; may adjust monthly dose (maintenance given deltoid or gluteal) Approx. equivalence: 3 mg oral: 39–78 mg 6 mg oral: 117 mg 12 mg oral: 234 mg	$$$$$
Paliperidone palmitate (Invega Trinza) 2015	Schizophrenia (only after at least 4 months of adequate treatment on Sustenna)	273, 410, 546, 819 mg prefilled syringes	No overlap	3 months	Based on previous monthly Sustenna dose: For 78 mg, give 273 mg Trinza For 117 mg, give 410 mg Trinza For 156 mg, give 546 mg Trinza For 234 mg, give 819 mg Trinza	Give same conversion dose of Trinza every 3 months; adjust if necessary per patient response	$$$$$
Paliperidone palmitate (Invega Hafyera) 2021	Schizophrenia (only after at least 4 months of adequate treatment on Sustenna or 3 months on Trinza)	1,092, 1,560 mg prefilled syringes	No overlap	6 months	Based on previous monthly Sustenna dose: For 156 mg, give 1,092 mg Hafyera For 234 mg, give 1,560 mg Hafyera Or based on 3-month Trinza dose: For 546 mg, give 1,092 mg Hafyera For 819 mg, give 1,560 mg Hafyera	Give same conversion dose of Hafyera every 6 months; adjust if necessary per patient response	$$$$$
Risperidone (Risperdal Consta) 2003	Schizophrenia Bipolar, manic/mixed (monotherapy or adjunct)	12.5, 25, 37.5, 50 mg vials	With usual oral dose for 3 weeks	2 weeks	Start at 25 mg Q2 weeks; adjust dose no more frequently than Q4 weeks as needed for response	Approx. equivalence: <4 mg/day oral: 25 mg 4–6 mg/day oral: 37.5 mg >6 mg/day oral: 50 mg Maximum dose: 50 mg Q2 weeks	$$$$$
Risperidone (Perseris) 2018	Schizophrenia	90, 120 mg	No overlap	Monthly	Start 90 or 120 mg SQ to abdomen monthly	Approx. equivalence: 90 mg monthly: 3 mg/day oral 120 mg monthly: 4 mg/day oral	$$$$$

¹brand discontinued; available as generic only

Anxiolytics and Hypnotics

ANXIOLYTICS

Anxiety is perhaps the most frequent symptom for which child psychiatrists are consulted. There are many medications to choose from, and clinicians all have their personal algorithms that vary depending on the situation. While selective serotonin reuptake inhibitors (SSRIs) are generally considered the mainstay medications for anxiety, it is important to consider other options, particularly because of SSRIs' potential for side effects. Here are some pros and cons of the major options.

Treating the core four: The first AACAP Clinical Practice Guideline, released in the fall of 2020, focused on anxiety disorders. It's worth a full read, but here's the bottom line: "AACAP suggests that combination treatment (CBT and an SSRI) could be offered preferentially over CBT alone or an SSRI alone to patients 6 to 18 years old with social anxiety, generalized anxiety, separation anxiety, or panic disorder."

Here are the main categories of medications that clinicians typically use to treat anxiety in children and adolescents:

- **Alpha-adrenergics:** Central alpha-agonists include the alpha-2 agonists guanfacine and clonidine, plus the alpha-1 antagonist prazosin. These medications are approved for use in hypertension, and some of them are approved for ADHD. They reduce sympathetic tone, resulting in a mild reduction in internal tension and vigilance that is often very helpful. They are also useful in reducing tics. Prazosin can be helpful for nightmares, particularly those associated with PTSD. Common side effects include dizziness and sedation. These medications often have associated tachyphylaxis (ie, rapid tolerance to the dose, resulting in a need for higher dose); however, this tends to abate after the first few weeks. Central alpha-agonists are associated with irritability, perhaps related to the sedation they create.

- **Beta-blockers:** The most commonly used beta-blocker in child psychiatry is propranolol. It is useful for performance anxiety and other situations in which reducing the physiological symptoms of anxiety (ie, rapid or pounding heartbeat) would be helpful. There has been recent interest in using propranolol to help autistic children become more comfortable with social situations. Common side effects include reduced blood pressure in teens and reduced exercise tolerance in children of all ages. Of note, fluoxetine can increase levels of propranolol, and if this leads to more tiredness, it may be mistaken as depression and lead to an unnecessary increase of the fluoxetine dose.

- **SSRIs:** SSRIs are the only FDA-approved medications for anxiety disorders in children, specifically fluoxetine, fluvoxamine, and sertraline for OCD. Beyond OCD, SSRIs have a broad research evidence base for anxiety in children and adolescents, including studies in generalized anxiety disorder (GAD), social phobia, and separation anxiety. In general, we recommend using a lower initial SSRI dose for patients with anxiety disorders, particularly panic disorder. The disadvantage of SSRIs is their substantial side effects, in particular behavioral activation, which can be mistaken for increased anxiety, ADHD, or oppositionality. Like adults, children and teens may also experience side effects such as amotivational syndrome, manic or hypomanic episodes, GI disturbances, and excessive sweating (the latter a possible harbinger of serotonergic syndrome).

- **Mirtazapine:** Mirtazapine is helpful for anxiety, depression, insomnia, poor appetite, and GI distress in adults. It may be appropriate for some kids, though pediatric data are mostly limited to kids with depression. Side effects include sedation and overeating.

- **Serotonin and norepinephrine reuptake inhibitors (SNRIs):** Except for OCD, for which SNRIs have less utility, these medications have similar uses as SSRIs. A distinct disadvantage of SNRIs is their tendency toward problems with physiological withdrawal. Of the SNRIs, duloxetine is the only agent with an FDA indication for GAD (for kids 7 and up). Venlafaxine showed superiority over placebo in studies of kids with social anxiety and GAD. As a group, the most recent AACAP Clinical Practice Guidelines cite SNRIs as less effective and having more side effects than SSRIs for social anxiety, GAD, panic disorder, separation anxiety, and specific phobias. Still, family history of a good outcome may count toward trying an SNRI.

- **Buspirone:** Buspirone may have some value in some children and teens with anxiety symptoms. While there are case reports of efficacy, there is one negative study for GAD. Buspirone may help in GAD, but it's unlikely to help in other anxiety disorders. It is relatively innocuous in terms of side effects.

- **Tricyclic antidepressants (TCAs):** In former days, TCAs were considered a panacea for children's "behavioral issues," used for anxiety, depression, insomnia, ADHD, and bedwetting. Concerns about cardiac dangers dampened enthusiasm; however, clomipramine remains frequently used for OCD when SSRIs or SNRIs fail. In addition, neurologists and others continue to use TCAs for migraine and other pain syndromes. ECGs are recommended at initiation and follow-up due to risks of arrhythmias, including the potentially deadly torsades de pointes. These medications must be kept securely locked away as they are extremely dangerous in overdose.

- **Anticonvulsants:** Anticonvulsants used in child psychiatry include gabapentin, pregabalin, valproate, carbamazepine, and oxcarbazepine. All of these are sometimes used for severe anxiety, though usually in the context of comorbid conditions such as mood disorders or developmental disorders. It is important to note that there have been some reports of gabapentin and pregabalin misuse, and this risk might guide clinical use with some patients and families.

- **Antipsychotics:** Antipsychotics are sometimes used for severe anxiety—usually, but not always, in combination with other medications. However, given the array of potential side effects (such as weight gain), there are usually better options.

- **Benzodiazepines:** Other than exceptionally controlled and rare use for specific phobias, surgical procedures, severe childhood schizophrenia, and catatonia, the risks of benzodiazepines in children and adolescents far outweigh the benefits. Common problems include interference in memory and learning, sedation, reduced motor coordination, and paradoxical agitation. If you do use them, we recommend those with relatively longer half-lives (such as lorazepam as opposed to alprazolam), using low doses, using them only briefly (for days, not weeks), staying alert to the risk for misuse and diversion, and using them in support of a comprehensive plan that, for chronic conditions, includes psychotherapy.

Discontinuing anxiolytics: The general treatment of most anxiety disorders has a couple of nearly equivalent paths, with therapy and medication fairly equal in efficacy and the combination a bit more effective. The better-studied therapies are usually cognitive-behavioral approaches lasting about eight to 12 weeks. What does that say about medication? Ideally, when you use medication for an anxiety disorder, the child or teen will also receive therapy that helps them to function as you ease down on the medication over several weeks or a couple of months. If your patient starts to have more difficulty as you reduce the dosage, you may need to redouble efforts at therapy.

Treating related conditions:

- **OCD:** After ruling out PANS/PANDAS, CBT is the main go-to approach for OCD. However, SSRIs can be very helpful, often at dosages far above what we might use for the core four anxiety disorders or for depression. When two trials of SSRIs fail, think about clomipramine (check ECG and lock the medication up for safety). If that doesn't work, consider trying mirtazapine, SNRIs, buspirone, or an antiepileptic (eg, topiramate) before you try adjunctive second-generation antipsychotics.

- **PTSD:** Begin with principles of trauma-informed care (ie, safety, choices, collaboration, trustworthiness, and empowerment). Our algorithm has examples of phrases to get you started. Trauma-informed CBT (TFCBT) is the next step for patients who can participate in it. For those who cannot (usually because of developmental differences or being too young), consider parent-child interaction therapy (PCIT) or other developmental relationship-based approaches. There are no medications with FDA-approved indications for PTSD; however, central alpha-agonists might reduce nightmares, and for increased heart rate you might try teaching breathing techniques or prescribing beta-blockers. If the child is still symptomatic, SSRIs such as fluoxetine, sertraline, or escitalopram might be helpful.

- **Severe agitation:** First-line treatment of agitation in children and teens should include exploring the reasons for the upset (eg, hungry, angry, lonely, tired [HALT] and all sorts of misunderstandings) and use of calm, quiet spaces, soft voices, hydration, and food. Address sensory overstimulation, especially for autistic youth, and stay present rather than ignoring the person. PO or sublingual medication is preferred over IM when feasible and is probably nearly as effective. When IM medication treatment is necessary, it is patterned after adult studies: IM olanzapine is probably more effective than IM ziprasidone. IM lorazepam can augment IM ziprasidone, but avoid using it with olanzapine due to the potential for cardiorespiratory depression.

- **Catatonia:** Failure to recognize catatonia leads to increased morbidity and potentially mortality. We do not want to contribute to a "fad," but catatonia may be more common than usually recognized, especially with use of antipsychotics and with autism. Keep catatonia in your differential, review the DSM-5 criteria, and get consultation if you are unsure, but act promptly if a patient is not eating, is aspirating, has severe autonomic instability, or has other potentially catastrophic symptoms. Treatment typically incudes: 1) discontinuing antipsychotics; 2) supportive care; 3) careful assertive use of lorazepam, possibly in much higher than usual dosages; and 4) ECT for life-threatening malignant catatonia.

HYPNOTICS

No meds to start. Sleep disorders, like anxiety disorders, are another area where non-pharmacological approaches should take clear precedence. Rule out sleep apnea either by history or perhaps using a sleep study, and then use cognitive behavioral therapy for insomnia (CBT-i) as a first-line treatment. While it is common to teach parents sleep hygiene measures, such as electronics restrictions, regular schedules, later-morning starts for teens, and regular exercise, these maneuvers typically fail because of cognitive and behavioral barriers that you can address with CBT-i. Sleep studies in young children can be challenging due to discomfort and issues of separation at night.

Sleep medications should be used only for brief periods of one or two weeks, then tapered over several days and discontinued. They should probably be restricted in infants and young children due to safety concerns including dependence, delirium, and in some cases death, the latter possibly by inadvertent overdose. The possible exception might be in cases of severe developmental challenges accompanied by persistent and truly intractable insomnia, or perhaps in rare instances of classic early childhood mania.

Some clinicians might try herbal remedies first. Chamomile tea, while mild, is a good first-line off-the-shelf product that goes well with the implementation of better sleep hygiene practices. Valerian, also mild, comes in capsules and is also often helpful, although it sometimes carries an unpleasant odor. While kava is sometimes listed as another "natural herbal" sleep remedy, many people have severe side effects, including intense dreams, oversedation, intoxication, and physiological dependence. Rare cases of hepatic failure have been reported but are likely due to contaminants, not kava itself.

When you must use medication, our order of medications is roughly the following:

- **Central alpha-agonists and antagonists:** Guanfacine and clonidine are often helpful for initiating sleep. Clonidine may last only a few hours and result in rebound insomnia. Prazosin, an alpha-antagonist, may help as well, especially in the setting of PTSD with nightmares.

- **Melatonin:** Melatonin, an endogenous sleep hormone, has come into regular use in kids despite mixed studies showing little efficacy and some showing rebound insomnia when discontinued. Early concerns about safety (eg, reports of seizures) have not persisted, so this medication is mostly seen as benign. Melatonin has a short half-life and may cause rebound waking at night, although long-acting preparations are now available. Some people report vivid dreaming when they use melatonin.

- **Ramelteon:** This potent melatonin receptor agonist typically requires several weeks to see benefits. Since teens often do not have patience for such a trial, it can be a tough sell for them. Its use in children is relatively rare as most opt for melatonin instead. Still, it is among the more benign sleep medications.

- **Antihistamines:** Diphenhydramine, doxylamine, cyproheptadine, and hydroxyzine are commonly used in both adults and children to induce sleep. All of these may cause delirium or disinhibition. They may be habit-forming and therefore should be used with care. Occasional reports of overdose deaths have also been reported. Recent questions about lifetime cumulative use of anticholinergic medications in adults with later risk for dementia may beg caution in use of diphenhydramine, particularly if there is a known increased lifetime risk of dementia (eg, in Down syndrome or with family history of dementia).

- **Sedating antidepressants:** These medications, including mirtazapine and imipramine, can be useful for helping children and adolescents to sleep. Both mirtazapine and imipramine may create daytime sedation. Mirtazapine contributes more to increase in appetite, and imipramine has more potential for cardiac arrhythmias (particularly in overdose). ECGs should be considered if there is any suspicion of cardiac risk or if dosages exceed any but the smallest available pills. Trazodone, another older antidepressant, is often used in adults with insomnia, although it is prone to cause more daytime cognitive clouding and carries a small risk of priapism. While it is sometimes used in children and adolescents as well, we tend to avoid it due to concerns about cognitive clouding and possible interference in school function, sports, driving, and other activities requiring coordination and clear thinking.

- **Benzodiazepine hypnotics:** We try to avoid benzodiazepines such as temazepam due to risks of rapid dependence, impairment of memory and motor function, and association with falls and motor vehicle accidents. However, benzos may be useful specifically for night terrors or intractable insomnia. In such cases, we recommend a medication with a medium half-life, such as lorazepam, to avoid rebound insomnia or morning grogginess; it should be prescribed in a short course as part of a comprehensive intervention plan. Lorazepam is the first-line, although off-label, treatment for catatonia, and in that circumstance may require higher-than-usual dosages.

- **Non-benzodiazepine hypnotics:** We also avoid zolpidem, zaleplon, and eszopiclone, partly for the failure of controlled studies of the z-drugs, as well as for the propensity of these medications to elicit parasomnolent activity. The incidence of sleepwalking, sleep-talking, and other behaviors is higher in children than adults and can include dangerous wandering. Our own direct knowledge of catastrophic events in adult patients—driving, cooking, unremembered deals on overnight flights, and in one case a completed suicide—leave us unlikely to prescribe these medications to children and adolescents despite their popularity and heavy marketing.

Anxiety Disorders Treatment Algorithm for Children and Adolescents

*Denotes off label

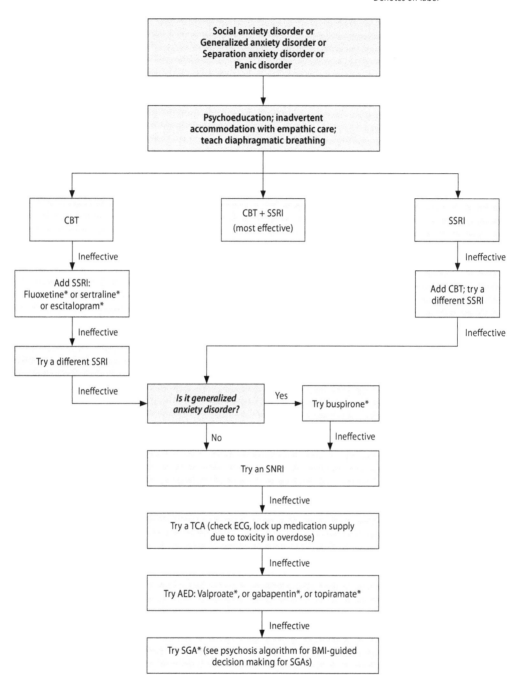

- Use non-pharmacologic approaches first when possible to help reduce use of medication
- See text and tables for specific age-related guidance
- If using antidepressants, discuss potential side effects including rare but possible increase in behavioral activation or suicidal thinking
- If using antipsychotics, check weight and labs (lipids, HbA1c, others as indicated) at baseline, 12 weeks, and yearly or sooner, AIMS at baseline and every 6 months or sooner, and consider ECG at baseline and yearly or sooner
- If stable for 2–6 months, consider gradual taper and discontinuation of medications

CARLAT PUBLISHING © 2023

Insomnia Treatment Algorithm for Children and Adolescents

*Denotes off label

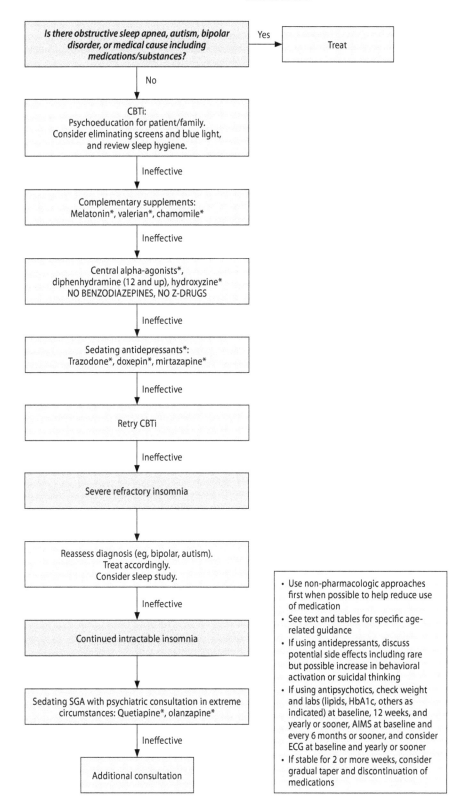

Is there obstructive sleep apnea, autism, bipolar disorder, or medical cause including medications/substances? → Yes → Treat

No ↓

CBTi:
Psychoeducation for patient/family. Consider eliminating screens and blue light, and review sleep hygiene.

Ineffective ↓

Complementary supplements:
Melatonin*, valerian*, chamomile*

Ineffective ↓

Central alpha-agonists*, diphenhydramine (12 and up), hydroxyzine*
NO BENZODIAZEPINES, NO Z-DRUGS

Ineffective ↓

Sedating antidepressants*:
Trazodone*, doxepin*, mirtazapine*

Ineffective ↓

Retry CBTi

Ineffective ↓

Severe refractory insomnia

↓

Reassess diagnosis (eg, bipolar, autism).
Treat accordingly.
Consider sleep study.

Ineffective ↓

Continued intractable insomnia

↓

Sedating SGA with psychiatric consultation in extreme circumstances: Quetiapine*, olanzapine*

Ineffective ↓

Additional consultation

- Use non-pharmacologic approaches first when possible to help reduce use of medication
- See text and tables for specific age-related guidance
- If using antidepressants, discuss potential side effects including rare but possible increase in behavioral activation or suicidal thinking
- If using antipsychotics, check weight and labs (lipids, HbA1c, others as indicated) at baseline, 12 weeks, and yearly or sooner, AIMS at baseline and every 6 months or sooner, and consider ECG at baseline and yearly or sooner
- If stable for 2 or more weeks, consider gradual taper and discontinuation of medications

Anxiolytics and Hypnotics

CARLAT PUBLISHING © 2023

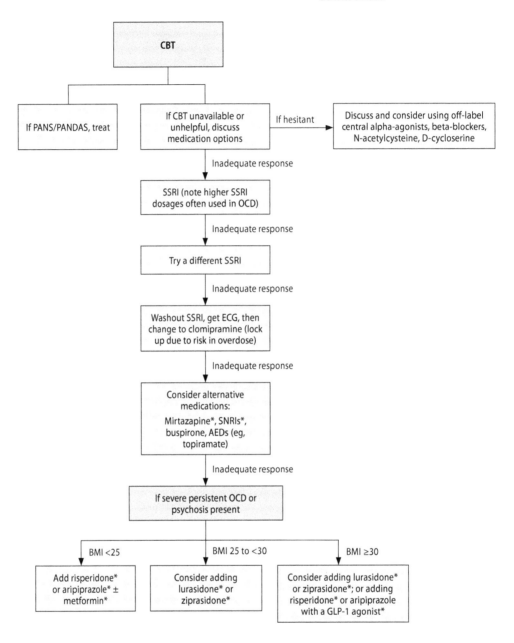

OCD Treatment Algorithm for Children and Adolescents

*Denotes off label

CBT

- If PANS/PANDAS, treat
- If CBT unavailable or unhelpful, discuss medication options
  - If hesitant → Discuss and consider using off-label central alpha-agonists, beta-blockers, N-acetylcysteine, D-cycloserine

↓ Inadequate response

SSRI (note higher SSRI dosages often used in OCD)

↓ Inadequate response

Try a different SSRI

↓ Inadequate response

Washout SSRI, get ECG, then change to clomipramine (lock up due to risk in overdose)

↓ Inadequate response

Consider alternative medications:

Mirtazapine*, SNRIs*, buspirone, AEDs (eg, topiramate)

↓ Inadequate response

If severe persistent OCD or psychosis present

- **BMI <25**: Add risperidone* or aripiprazole* ± metformin*
- **BMI 25 to <30**: Consider adding lurasidone* or ziprasidone*
- **BMI ≥30**: Consider adding lurasidone* or ziprasidone*; or adding risperidone* or aripiprazole with a GLP-1 agonist*

- Use non-pharmacologic approaches first when possible to help reduce use of medication
- See text and tables for specific age-related guidance
- If using antidepressants, discuss potential side effects including rare but possible increase in behavioral activation or suicidal thinking
- If using antipsychotics, check weight and labs (lipids, HbA1c, others as indicated) at baseline, 12 weeks, and yearly or sooner, AIMS at baseline and every 6 months or sooner, and consider ECG at baseline and yearly or sooner
- If stable for 3–12 months, consider gradual taper and discontinuation of medications

PTSD Treatment Algorithm for Children and Adolescents

*Denotes off label

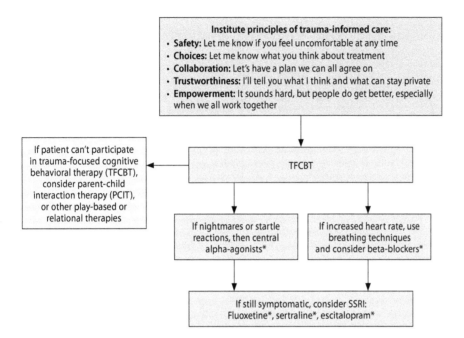

Institute principles of trauma-informed care:
- **Safety:** Let me know if you feel uncomfortable at any time
- **Choices:** Let me know what you think about treatment
- **Collaboration:** Let's have a plan we can all agree on
- **Trustworthiness:** I'll tell you what I think and what can stay private
- **Empowerment:** It sounds hard, but people do get better, especially when we all work together

TFCBT

If patient can't participate in trauma-focused cognitive behavioral therapy (TFCBT), consider parent-child interaction therapy (PCIT), or other play-based or relational therapies

If nightmares or startle reactions, then central alpha-agonists*

If increased heart rate, use breathing techniques and consider beta-blockers*

If still symptomatic, consider SSRI: Fluoxetine*, sertraline*, escitalopram*

- Use non-pharmacologic approaches first when possible to help reduce use of medication
- See text and tables for specific age-related guidance
- If using antidepressants, discuss potential side effects including rare but possible increase in behavioral activation or suicidal thinking
- If stable for 3 months, consider slow taper and discontinuation of medications

CARLAT PUBLISHING © 2023

Anxiolytics and Hypnotics

*Denotes off label

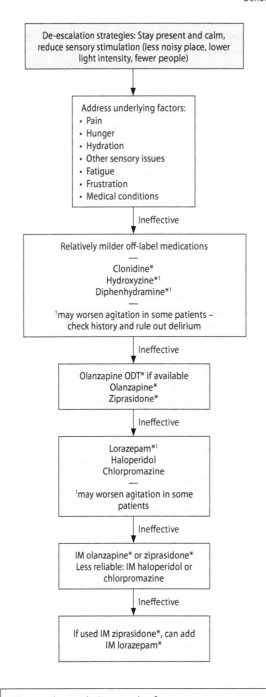

De-escalation strategies: Stay present and calm,
reduce sensory stimulation (less noisy place, lower
light intensity, fewer people)

Address underlying factors:
- Pain
- Hunger
- Hydration
- Other sensory issues
- Fatigue
- Frustration
- Medical conditions

Ineffective

Relatively milder off-label medications
—
Clonidine*
Hydroxyzine*[1]
Diphenhydramine*[1]
—
[1]may worsen agitation in some patients –
check history and rule out delirium

Ineffective

Olanzapine ODT* if available
Olanzapine*
Ziprasidone*

Ineffective

Lorazepam*[1]
Haloperidol
Chlorpromazine
—
[1]may worsen agitation in some
patients

Ineffective

IM olanzapine* or ziprasidone*
Less reliable: IM haloperidol or
chlorpromazine

Ineffective

If used IM ziprasidone*, can add
IM lorazepam*

- Use non-pharmacologic approaches first
- See text for age ranges for medications
- Monitor ECG and BP when using antipsychotics in this situation
- Watch for extrapyramidal symptions including dystonia

Catatonia Treatment Algorithm for Children and Adolescents

*Denotes off label

Carefully clarify diagnosis of catatonia separate from others (eg, autism, psychosis, bipolar disorder, major depression)

Life-threatening symptoms?
(eg, respiratory, dysphagia with risk of aspiration, NMS)
— Yes → ECT ASAP for malignant catatonia
No ↓

Is patient taking antipsychotic medications?
— Yes → Discontinue antipsychotic medications
No ↓

Non-pharmacological care:
eg, psycho-ecological model;
www.tinyurl.com/tvnejk6u
• Reduce stress
• Keep active
↓

Lorazepam* 0.5 mg PO TID.
Titrate by 0.5 mg PO TID every 2–3 days as needed to treat symptoms.
Maximum 8 mg PO TID. Monitor respiratory rate and PO2.
↓

Co-occurring psychosis?
— Yes → Careful rechallenge with antipsychotic treatment for psychosis
No ↓

Stable for 3 months?
No ↓

Consider ECT, or increased ECT

- Use non-pharmacologic approaches first when possible to help reduce use of medication
- See text and tables for specific age-related guidance
- If using antipsychotics, check weight and labs (lipids, HbA1c, others as indicated) at baseline, 12 weeks, and yearly or sooner, AIMS at baseline and every 6 months or sooner, and consider ECG at baseline and yearly or sooner
- If stable for 3 months, consider gradual taper and discontinuation of medications, ECT

CARLAT PUBLISHING © 2023

Anxiolytics and Hypnotics

TABLE 9: Anxiolytics and Hypnotics

Generic Name (Brand Name) Year FDA Approved *[G] denotes generic availability*	Relevant FDA Indication(s) (Pediatric indications in bold)	Available Strengths (mg)	Onset of Action (oral)[2]	Half-Life (hours)	Duration of Action (hours)	Usual Pediatric Dosage Range (starting–max) (mg)	Comments
Alprazolam [G] (Xanax, Xanax XR) 1981	GAD Panic disorder	Tablet: 0.25, 0.5, 1, 2 ER tablet: 0.5, 1, 2, 3 ODT: 0.25, 0.5, 1, 2 Liquid: 1 mg/mL	30 min (IR, ODT); 1–2 hrs (XR)	11–16	3–4 (IR) 10 (XR)	0.375–3.5 mg/day divided TID	NOT RECOMMENDED. Very limited data showing no benefit over placebo in GAD or school refusal/separation anxiety.
Buspirone [G] (BuSpar[1]) 1986	GAD	Tablet: 5, 7.5, 10, 15, 30	1–2 wks+	2–3	N/A	5–20 TID	Very limited data showing no benefit over placebo in GAD.
Clomipramine [G] (Anafranil) 1989	**OCD (10+ yrs)**	25, 50, 75	1–2 wks+	32	N/A	25–200 QHS	Use for OCD if SSRI fails or is not tolerated.
Clonazepam [G] (Klonopin, Klonopin Wafers[1]) 1975	**Absence, petit mal, akinetic, and myoclonic seizures (myoclonia) (≤10 yrs)** Panic disorder; insomnia (off label)	Tablet: 0.5, 1, 2 ODT: 0.125, 0.25, 0.5, 1, 2	1 hr	20–80	4–8	0.125–1 BID	NOT RECOMMENDED. Very limited data showing no benefit over placebo in GAD or social phobia.
Clonidine [G] (Catapres) 1974	**ER (Kapvay) approved for ADHD (6–17 yrs);** anxiety (off label)	IR: 0.1, 0.2, 0.3 ER: 0.1, 0.2	1 hr	12–16	4–6	0.05–0.4 QHS or divided doses	Used especially when comorbid ADHD or tics; do not stop an ongoing dosage abruptly (rebound hypertension).
Diazepam [G] (Valium, Diastat) 1963	**Seizures and spasm (infants+, but neonate off label);** GAD; alcohol withdrawal; **anxiety (short term) (0.5+ yrs)**	Tablet: 2, 5, 10 Liquid: 5 mg/5 mL, 5 mg/mL Injection: 5 mg/mL Rectal gel: 2.5, 5, 7.5, 10, 12.5, 15, 17.5, 20	30 min	>100	4–6	0.04–0.2 mg/kg Q2–4h PRN (0.5–12 yrs) 2–10 mg BID–QID (≥13 yrs)	NOT RECOMMENDED for anxiety or insomnia. Typically used as one-time dose in emergency, dental, or seizure settings.
Diphenhydramine [G] (Benadryl, others) 1946 Available OTC and Rx	**Insomnia (12+ yrs); allergy (20+ lbs); motion sickness (6+ yrs)**	Capsule: 25, 50 Tablet: 25 Liquid: 12.5 mg/mL	1 hr	3.5–9	4–6	6.25–50 QHS	Some benefit in pediatric patients; caution for paradoxical reaction.
Doxepin [G] (Silenor, Sinequan) 2020/1969	**Insomnia (sleep maintenance)**	Tablet: 3, 6 Capsule: 10, 25, 50, 75, 100, 150 Liquid: 10 mg/mL	1 hr	15	4–6	3–50 QHS	Helpful for sleep; caution for daytime sedation, cardiac arrhythmias.
Doxylamine [G] (Unisom, others) 1978 Available OTC and Rx	**Nighttime sleep aid (12+ yrs); rhinitis (2+ yrs)**	Tablet: 25	1 hr	10	4–6	6.25–50 QHS	Some benefit in pediatric patients; caution for paradoxical reaction.

Generic Name (Brand Name) Year FDA Approved [G] denotes generic availability	Relevant FDA Indication(s) (Pediatric indications in bold)	Available Strengths (mg)	Onset of Action (oral)[2]	Half-Life (hours)	Duration of Action (hours)	Usual Pediatric Dosage Range (starting–max) (mg)	Comments
Eszopiclone [G] (Lunesta) 2004	Insomnia (sleep onset and sleep maintenance)	Tablet: 1, 2, 3	30 min	6	6–8	1–3 QHS	NOT RECOMMENDED. No benefit in pediatric patients.
Gabapentin [G] (Neurontin) 1993	Anxiety **Seizures (3+ yrs)**	Capsule: 100, 300, 400 Tablet: 600, 800 Oral solution: 50 mg/mL ER tablet: 300, 600	1–2 hrs	5–7	6–8	100 QHS–300 TID	Very limited data; reserve for severe anxiety or comorbidity; caution regarding misuse.
Guanfacine IR [G] (Tenex) 1986	ADHD (only ER approved)	1, 2	1 hr	13–14	N/A	0.5–4 QD (do not increase faster than 1 mg/wk)	Very limited data suggesting improvement in generalized, separation, or social anxiety disorder; do not stop abruptly (rebound hypertension); not a 1:1 conversion from IR; do not give with high-fat meals; use especially when comorbid ADHD.
Guanfacine ER [G] (Intuniv) 2009	**ADHD (6–17 yrs)**	1, 2, 3, 4	1–2 hrs	13–14	N/A	1–4 QD (do not increase faster than 1 mg/wk) (adolescents 7 mg/day max)	
Hydroxyzine [G] (Atarax, Vistaril) 1956	**Anxiety (6+ yrs); pruritis (<6 yrs by weight)**	Capsule: 25, 50, 100 Tablet: 10, 25, 50 Liquid: 10 mg/5 mL Injection: 25 mg/mL, 50 mg/mL	1 hr	20–25	4–6	12.5–100 QHS	Commonly used and helpful for inducing sleep but may cause grogginess, delirium, or disinhibition.
Imipramine [G] Tofranil brand discontinued; generic only 1984	MDD; **nocturnal enuresis (6+ yrs)**	10, 25, 50, 75, 100, 125, 150	1–2 wks+	11–25	N/A	10–100 QHS	May be helpful for sleep; caution for daytime sedation, cardiac arrhythmias.
Lorazepam [G] (Ativan, Loreev XR) 1977	GAD; insomnia (off label); **anxiety (short term) (12+ yrs)**	Tablet: 0.5, 1, 2 ER capsule: 1, 2, 3 Liquid: 2 mg/mL Injection: 2 mg/mL, 4 mg/mL	30–60 min	10–20	4–6	0.05 mg/kg Q4–8h PRN; max 2 mg/dose	NOT RECOMMENDED. No benefit in pediatric patients, except in catatonia.
Mirtazapine [G] (Remeron) 1996	MDD	Tablet: 7.5, 15, 30, 45 ODT: 15, 30, 45	1–2 wks+	20–40	N/A	7.5–45 QHS	May be helpful for sleep; caution for daytime sedation, increased appetite.
Prazosin [G] (Minipress) 1976	PTSD (off label)	Capsule: 1, 2, 5	1–2 hrs	2–3	4–6	1–10 mg/day QHS or divided BID	Minimal data but may consider in PTSD-associated nightmares or sleep disturbances; monitor BP.
Pregabalin [G] (Lyrica) 2004	Anxiety (off label) Neuropathic pain; fibromyalgia; seizures	Capsule: 25, 50, 75, 100, 200, 225, 300 Oral solution: 20 mg/mL	1–2 hrs	6	8–12	75–300 QHS	Very limited data; reserve for severe anxiety or comorbidity; caution regarding misuse.
Propranolol [G] (Inderal) 1973	Performance anxiety, tremor (off label)	Tablet: 10, 20, 40, 60, 80	60 min	3–6	4–6	<35 kg: 10–20 mg TID ≥35 kg: 20–40 mg TID	Effective for performance anxiety but no data in kids.

Generic Name (Brand Name) Year FDA Approved [G] denotes generic availability	Relevant FDA Indication(s) (Pediatric indications in bold)	Available Strengths (mg)	Onset of Action (oral)[2]	Half-Life (hours)	Duration of Action (hours)	Usual Pediatric Dosage Range (starting–max) (mg)	Comments
Ramelteon (Rozerem) 2005	Insomnia (sleep onset)	Tablet: 8	30 min	1–2.6	Unknown	8 QHS	Less risky hypnotic but no data in kids.
Temazepam [G] (Restoril) 1981	Insomnia (short term)	Capsule: 7.5, 15, 22.5, 30	30–60 min	9–18	4–6	7.5–30 QHS	NOT RECOMMENDED. No benefit in pediatric patients.
Trazodone [G] (Desyrel[3], Oleptro[3]) 1981/2010	Depression Insomnia (off label)	Tablet: 50, 100, 150, 300 ER tablet: 150, 300	1 hr	7–10	Unknown	25–200 QHS	Used especially in kids with depression or anxiety.
Triazolam [G] (Halcion) 1982	Insomnia (short term)	Tablet: 0.125, 0.25	15–30 min	1.5–5.5	Unknown	0.125–0.5 QHS	NOT RECOMMENDED. No benefit in pediatric patients.
Zaleplon [G] (Sonata) 1999	Insomnia (short term, sleep onset)	Capsule: 5, 10	30 min	1	4	10–20 QHS	NOT RECOMMENDED. No benefit in pediatric patients.
Zolpidem [G] (Ambien, Ambien CR, Edluar, Zolpimist) 1992 Generic not available for Zolpimist or Edluar SL	Insomnia (IR: short term, sleep onset; CR: sleep onset and maintenance)	Tablet: 5, 10 ER tablet: 6.25, 12.5 SL tablet: 5, 10 Oral spray: 5 mg/spray	30 min	2.5–3	6–8	10, 12.5 CR (5, 6.25 in women)	NOT RECOMMENDED. No benefit in pediatric patients.
Zolpidem low dose (Intermezzo) [G] 2011	Difficulty falling asleep after middle-of-the-night awakening	SL tablet: 1.75, 3.5	30 min	2.5	4	1.75 women; 3.5 men	NOT RECOMMENDED. No benefit in pediatric patients.

[1] For approximate benzodiazepine dose equivalencies, refer to Table 9.1

[2] Onset and duration vary from person to person, dose to dose, and preparation to preparation

[3] Brand discontinued; available as generic only

TABLE 9.1: Benzodiazepine Dosage Equivalencies

As noted in the preceding pages, benzodiazepines are generally not recommended for kids. When used, we generally stick to lorazepam or clonazepam. Lorazepam is a first-line (but off-label) treatment for catatonia. We've provided here a table of equivalencies for those cases where you may need to switch a child over to another benzodiazepine.

Benzodiazepine	Approximate Equivalent Dosage (mg)
Alprazolam (Xanax)	0.5
Chlordiazepoxide (Librium)	25
Clonazepam (Klonopin)	0.25–0.5
Clorazepate (Tranxene)	7.5
Diazepam (Valium)	5
Estazolam (Prosom)	1
Flurazepam (Dalmane)	15
Lorazepam (Ativan)	1
Oxazepam (Serax)	15
Quazepam (Doral)	15
Temazepam (Restoril)	15
Triazolam (Halcion)	0.25

Anxiolytics and Hypnotics

ANTIHISTAMINES (Diphenhydramine, Doxylamine, Hydroxyzine) Fact Sheet [G]

BOTTOM LINE:
Antihistamines can be effective sleepers for some kids and are the most prescribed by pediatricians, although some patients may experience too much grogginess ("hangover") in the morning or a paradoxical excitation. Good option to keep in your bag of tricks due to experience in kids and low risk of tolerance, dependence, or abuse.

PEDIATRIC FDA INDICATIONS:
- Diphenhydramine: **Insomnia** (12–17 years); allergies (20+ lbs); motion sickness (6+ years).
- Doxylamine: **Insomnia** (12+ years); rhinitis (12+ years).
- Hydroxyzine: **Anxiety** (6–17 years); pruritis (<6 years by weight).

ADULT FDA INDICATIONS:
Insomnia; allergies; motion sickness; anti-Parkinsonism.

OFF-LABEL USES:
EPS; nausea and vomiting (morning sickness).

DOSAGE FORMS:
- Diphenhydramine (G): Tablets, chewable tablets, caplets, capsules, and oral solutions, varies by brand: 25 mg, 50 mg. Available as Benadryl, Compoz, Nytol, Simply Sleep, Sleep-Eze, Sominex, Unisom SleepGels, Unisom SleepMelts, and generic.
- Doxylamine (G): Tablets: 25 mg. Available as NyQuil, Unisom SleepTabs, and generic.
- Hydroxyzine (G): Capsules: 25, 50, 100 mg; tablets: 10, 25, 50 mg; liquid: 10 mg/5 mL; injectable: 25 mg/mL, 50 mg/mL. Available as Atarax, Vistaril, and generic.

PEDIATRIC DOSAGE GUIDANCE:
- Diphenhydramine: Start 25 mg (use 12.5 mg in kids 6–11 years or 6.25 mg in kids 2–5 years) 30 minutes before bedtime. The dose required to induce sleep can be as low as 6.25 mg, but usual dose is 25 mg. Some older kids may require 50 mg at bedtime.
- Doxylamine: For insomnia in children 12+ years: 25 mg given 30 minutes before bedtime.
- Hydroxyzine: For children <6 years: 50 mg/day divided or 2 mg/kg/day divided every six to eight hours, or 15 mg/m^2/day given in divided doses; for children ≥6 years: 50–100 mg/day divided, or 2 mg/kg/day divided every six to eight hours.

MONITORING: No specific monitoring of note.

COST: $

SIDE EFFECTS:
- Most common: Dry mouth, ataxia, urinary retention, constipation, drowsiness, memory problems.
- Serious but rare: Blurred vision, tachycardia.

MECHANISM, PHARMACOKINETICS, AND DRUG INTERACTIONS:
- Histamine H1 antagonist.
- Metabolized by liver, primarily CYP2D6; t ½: for diphenhydramine, 3.5–9 hours; for doxylamine, 10 hours (12–15 hours in elderly); for hydroxyzine, 20–25 hours.
- Avoid use with other antihistamines or anticholinergics (additive effects).

EVIDENCE AND CLINICAL PEARLS:
- Controlled studies of diphenhydramine and placebo have reported mixed results. Two found it no better than placebo for sleep quality and maintenance in infants, children, and adolescents, while the third found improvement in sleep initiation and maintenance compared to placebo. One study in babies 6–15 months found diphenhydramine no better than placebo.
- These antihistamines non-selectively antagonize central and peripheral histamine H1 receptors. They also have secondary anticholinergic effects, which can cause side effects including dry mouth and urinary retention, as well as cognitive impairment in susceptible populations. Some kids may experience a paradoxical excitation.
- Tolerance may develop over time, necessitating use of higher doses. Best used as short-term sleep aid.
- Be aware that anticholinergic drugs are often used to treat or prevent EPS in patients taking antipsychotics; diphenhydramine is often chosen and dosed at night to take advantage of its sedative effect.

FUN FACT:
The name NyQuil is a portmanteau of "night" and "tranquil."

BUSPIRONE (BuSpar) Fact Sheet [G]

BOTTOM LINE:
Despite the lack of large randomized controlled data to support first-line use, buspirone may be used adjunctively in kids who exhibit partial response to first-line therapies for anxiety (SSRI, SNRI), without the sedation and abuse potential burden of benzodiazepines.

PEDIATRIC FDA INDICATIONS:
None.

ADULT FDA INDICATIONS:
GAD.

OFF-LABEL USES:
Treatment-resistant depression; anxiety symptoms in depression.

DOSAGE FORMS:
Tablets (G): 5 mg (scored), 7.5 mg (scored), 10 mg (scored), 15 mg (scored), 30 mg (scored).

PEDIATRIC DOSAGE GUIDANCE:
- No guidance on dosing in children and adolescents.
- Adult dosing: Start 7.5 mg BID or 5 mg TID; increase by increments of 5 mg/day every two to three days to target dose 20–30 mg/day divided BID–TID; max 20 mg TID.

MONITORING: No specific monitoring of note.

COST: $

SIDE EFFECTS:
Most common: Dizziness, nervousness, nausea, headache, jitteriness.

MECHANISM, PHARMACOKINETICS, AND DRUG INTERACTIONS:
- Serotonin 5HT1A receptor partial agonist.
- Metabolized primarily through CYP3A4; t ½: 2–3 hours.
- Avoid use with MAOIs; caution with serotonergic agents due to additive effects and risk for serotonin syndrome. Caution with CYP3A4 inhibitors or inducers as they may affect buspirone serum levels; adjust dose.

EVIDENCE AND CLINICAL PEARLS:
- Although very well tolerated, randomized placebo-controlled data found buspirone 15–60 mg/day to be no better than placebo in kids 6–17 years with GAD.
- Similar to antidepressants, buspirone requires one to two weeks for onset of therapeutic effects, with full effects occurring over several weeks, and offers no "as-needed" benefits.
- Non-sedating, non-habit-forming alternative to benzodiazepines for anxiety, but minimal efficacy data in kids show it may be no better than placebo.

FUN FACT:
Other psychotropic agents with 5HT1A partial agonist effects include aripiprazole, ziprasidone, and vilazodone.

Anxiolytics and Hypnotics

CLONAZEPAM (Klonopin) Fact Sheet [G]

BOTTOM LINE:
Due to the lack of large randomized controlled data to support its use and the potential for side effects, clonazepam should be avoided. If you decide to use it, keep it very short term and deploy it adjunctively in kids who exhibit only partial response to first-line therapies (SSRI, SNRI) or have severe anxiety.

PEDIATRIC FDA INDICATIONS:
Seizure disorders.

ADULT FDA INDICATIONS:
Seizure disorders; panic disorder.

OFF-LABEL USES:
Other anxiety disorders; insomnia; acute mania or psychosis; catatonia.

DOSAGE FORMS:
• **Tablets (G):** 0.5 mg (scored), 1 mg (scored), 2 mg (scored).
• **Orally disintegrating tablets (G):** 0.125 mg, 0.25 mg, 0.5 mg, 1 mg, 2 mg.

PEDIATRIC DOSAGE GUIDANCE:
• Minimal guidance on dosing in children and adolescents.
• Start 0.125–0.25 mg daily, increase by 0.125–0.25 mg/day increments as needed to response; max dose 2 mg/day.
• Dose varies based on patient characteristics (eg, age) and tolerance to benzodiazepines.

MONITORING: No specific monitoring of note.

COST: $

SIDE EFFECTS:
• Most common: Somnolence, daytime grogginess, confusion, ataxia.
• Serious but rare: Anterograde amnesia, increased fall risk, paradoxical reaction (irritability, agitation); respiratory depression (avoid in patients with sleep apnea or on opioids).

MECHANISM, PHARMACOKINETICS, AND DRUG INTERACTIONS:
• Binds to benzodiazepine receptors to enhance GABA effects.
• Metabolized primarily through CYP3A4; t ½: 20–80 hours.
• Avoid concomitant use with other CNS depressants, including alcohol and opioids (additive effects). Potent CYP3A4 inhibitors (eg, fluvoxamine, erythromycin) may increase clonazepam levels; CYP3A4 inducers (eg, carbamazepine) may decrease clonazepam levels.

EVIDENCE AND CLINICAL PEARLS:
• Double-blind placebo-controlled data found no benefit over placebo in 15 kids (7–13 years) with GAD or social phobia. Common side effects included irritability, drowsiness, and oppositional behavior.
• C-IV controlled substance.
• High-potency, long-acting benzodiazepine with active metabolites that may accumulate.
• Withdrawal effects may not be seen until three to five days after abrupt discontinuation and may last 10–14 days due to long half-life and active metabolites.
• Full effects of a particular dose may not be evident for a few days since active metabolites will accumulate with continual use (versus PRN use). Wait several days before increasing dose if patient is taking clonazepam regularly.

FUN FACT:
Klonopin tablets (or "K-pins") have a street value of $2–$5 per tablet, depending on dose and geographic region.

LORAZEPAM (Ativan) Fact Sheet [G]

BOTTOM LINE:
Benzodiazepines are generally only appropriate for use before procedures. Lorazepam probably has less risk of misuse than others. Lorazepam is also the first-line, but off-label, treatment for catatonia.

PEDIATRIC FDA INDICATIONS:
None.

ADULT FDA INDICATIONS:
GAD; status epilepticus (IV route).

OFF-LABEL USES:
Other anxiety disorders; insomnia; acute mania or psychosis; catatonia; preoperative sedation; chemo-related nausea/vomiting.

DOSAGE FORMS:
- **Tablets (G):** 0.5 mg (scored), 1 mg (scored), 2 mg (scored).
- **ER capsules (Loreev XR):** 1 mg, 2 mg, 3 mg.
- **Oral concentrate (G):** 2 mg/mL.
- **Injection (G):** 2 mg/mL, 4 mg/mL.

PEDIATRIC DOSAGE GUIDANCE:
- Anxiety: 0.05 mg/kg Q4–8h PRN; max 2 mg/dose.
- ER capsules for patients taking stable, evenly divided TID dosing with IR; to be taken once daily in morning. No data to support use in children.
- Insomnia (off-label use): Start 0.25–1 mg QHS, 20–30 minutes before bedtime; max 2 mg nightly.
- Catatonia: Start 0.5 mg TID, increase by 0.5 mg TID every two to three days based on response. While dosages of up to 8 mg TID have reportedly been required, and paradoxically to relieve respiratory depression, we recommend using extreme caution, an abundance of physiological monitoring, and continuing consultation in cases of severe catatonia.

MONITORING: No specific monitoring of note.

COST: $; Loreev XR: $$$$

SIDE EFFECTS:
- Most common: Somnolence, dizziness, weakness, ataxia.
- Serious but rare: Anterograde amnesia, increased fall risk, paradoxical reaction (irritability, agitation); respiratory depression (avoid in patients with sleep apnea or on opioids).

MECHANISM, PHARMACOKINETICS, AND DRUG INTERACTIONS:
- Binds to benzodiazepine receptors to enhance GABA effects.
- Metabolism primarily hepatic (non-CYP450) to inactive compounds; t ½: 10–20 hours.
- Avoid concomitant use with other CNS depressants, including alcohol and opioids (additive effects). No risk for CYP450 drug interactions.

EVIDENCE AND CLINICAL PEARLS:
- There are no pediatric studies in anxiety disorders. Evidence is mainly for pre-procedure single-dose use.
- C-IV controlled substance.
- Lorazepam does not have a long half-life or active metabolites that could accumulate, and it poses no CYP450 drug interaction risk.
- Withdrawal symptoms are usually seen on the first day after abrupt discontinuation and last five to seven days in patients receiving benzodiazepines with short to intermediate half-lives, such as lorazepam. A gradual taper is highly recommended, particularly if prolonged treatment on a high dose.
- Tolerance to sedative effect may develop within two to four weeks of use, and benzodiazepines affect the normal sleep architecture; thus, long-term use is discouraged.

FUN FACT:
Early Ativan marketing efforts included clever direct-to-consumer advertising campaigns. These included: "Now it can be yours—the Ativan experience" in 1977 and "In a world where certainties are few . . . no wonder Ativan is prescribed by so many caring clinicians" in 1987.

PRAZOSIN (Minipress) Fact Sheet [G]

BOTTOM LINE:
Although there are only minimal data, consider prazosin for PTSD in kids, especially for PTSD-associated sleep disturbances and nightmares, but monitor BP.

PEDIATRIC FDA INDICATIONS:
None.

ADULT FDA INDICATIONS:
Hypertension.

OFF-LABEL USES:
PTSD; alcohol use disorder.

DOSAGE FORMS:
Capsules (G): 1 mg, 2 mg, 5 mg.

PEDIATRIC DOSAGE GUIDANCE:
- PTSD (off-label): Doses studied are 0.02–0.3 mg/kg given at bedtime; titrate dose slowly to minimize possibility of "first-dose" orthostatic hypotension. Start 1 mg QHS x3 days, increase slowly based on response. Target 1–5 mg/day; doses up to 15 mg daily studied in adults.
- May dose-divide BID to target daytime PTSD-associated arousal symptoms.

MONITORING: BP.

COST: $

SIDE EFFECTS:
- Most common: Somnolence, dizziness, headache, weakness.
- Serious but rare: Orthostasis and syncope; prolonged erections and priapism have been reported.

MECHANISM, PHARMACOKINETICS, AND DRUG INTERACTIONS:
- Alpha-1 adrenergic receptor antagonist.
- Metabolism primarily hepatic (non-CYP450); t ½: 2–3 hours.
- Caution with other antihypertensive agents, diuretics, and PDE5 inhibitors (eg, Viagra) that may have additive hypotensive effects.

EVIDENCE AND CLINICAL PEARLS:
- Initial studies in adults showed improvement in trauma-related nightmares and sleep quality when dosed at bedtime. Subsequent randomized controlled trials have shown positive effects on daytime PTSD symptoms also when dosed BID.
- A retrospective chart review of 34 kids (5–18 years) with PTSD suggested prazosin is well tolerated and associated with improvements in nightmares and sleep.
- Prazosin failed to work in a more recent controlled trial of military veterans with chronic PTSD. This was the largest study to date on this drug, but it had some flaws: The placebo rate was unusually high, and the investigators may have enriched their sample with patients who were less likely to respond to prazosin.

FUN FACT:
Prazosin is an effective drug for kids in the treatment of serious scorpion envenomations with significant sympathetic symptoms.

PROPRANOLOL (Inderal) Fact Sheet [G]

BOTTOM LINE:
May be effective and safe for use in performance anxiety, particularly when the sedating or cognitive side effects of benzos could interfere with an individual's performance, but there are no data in kids.

PEDIATRIC FDA INDICATIONS:
None.

ADULT FDA INDICATIONS:
Hypertension; angina; post-MI cardioprotection; atrial fibrillation; migraine prophylaxis; essential tremor.

OFF-LABEL USES:
Performance anxiety; tremor due to medication side effects (especially lithium); akathisia.

DOSAGE FORMS:
Tablets (G): 10 mg, 20 mg, 40 mg, 60 mg, 80 mg (all scored).

PEDIATRIC DOSAGE GUIDANCE:
- Minimal guidance on dosing in children and adolescents.
- Start 5–10 mg QD, increase by 5 mg/day increments as needed to response; max dose 20 mg/day. May divide dose BID.
- Performance anxiety (off-label use): Give 10 mg about 60 minutes prior to performance; usual effective dose for most is 10–20 mg.
- Medication-induced tremor: Start 10 mg BID as needed, can go up to 30–120 mg daily in two or three divided doses. Can also use Inderal LA, long-acting version of propranolol, 60–80 mg once a day.

MONITORING: BP/P.

COST: $

SIDE EFFECTS:
- Most common: Dizziness, fatigue, bradycardia, hypotension.
- Theoretically may exacerbate asthma symptoms, although studies are equivocal.

MECHANISM, PHARMACOKINETICS, AND DRUG INTERACTIONS:
- Non-selective beta-1 and beta-2 adrenergic receptor antagonist.
- Metabolized primarily through CYP2D6, also CYP1A2 and CYP2C19; t ½: 3–6 hours. Be careful about inadvertent increase with fluoxetine leading to fatigue that might be misinterpreted as increased depression.
- Caution with other antihypertensives (additive effects). CYP2D6 inhibitors, and CYP1A2 and CYP2C19 inhibitors or inducers, may affect propranolol levels.

EVIDENCE AND CLINICAL PEARLS:
- No data for treating anxiety in children.
- With beta-blockade, propranolol reduces some of the somatic symptoms of anxiety (tremor, sweating, flushing, tachycardia).

FUN FACT:
The list of notable people who suffer or have suffered from performance anxiety or stage fright is long. It includes Barbra Streisand, Carly Simon, Van Morrison, Frédéric Chopin, Renée Fleming, Jay Mohr, Hugh Grant, Laurence Olivier, Mahatma Gandhi, and Thomas Jefferson, among others.

RAMELTEON (Rozerem) Fact Sheet [G]

BOTTOM LINE:
Ramelteon is a melatonin receptor agonist with no data in pediatric patients. In adults, and compared to other hypnotics, ramelteon poses a lower risk for respiratory depression and hangover effect (morning grogginess) but takes longer to take effect. Also consider that over-the-counter melatonin (which ramelteon mimics) may do the same job, possibly at a lower price.

PEDIATRIC FDA INDICATIONS:
None.

ADULT FDA INDICATIONS:
Insomnia (sleep onset).

OFF-LABEL USES:
Jet lag; shift-work sleep disorder.

DOSAGE FORMS:
Tablets (G): 8 mg.

DOSAGE GUIDANCE:
- Minimal guidance on dosing in children and adolescents.
- Start, target, and maximum dose 8 mg QHS, 30 minutes before bedtime. Avoid administering with high-fat meal (delays therapeutic effect by 45 minutes).

MONITORING: No routine monitoring recommended unless clinical picture warrants.

COST: $$

SIDE EFFECTS:
- Most common: Headache, somnolence, fatigue, dizziness, nausea.
- Serious but rare: Anaphylaxis, angioedema, complex sleep-related behavior (sleep driving, cooking, eating, phone calls), increased prolactin, abnormal cortisol or testosterone levels.

MECHANISM, PHARMACOKINETICS, AND DRUG INTERACTIONS:
- Melatonin-1 and melatonin-2 receptor agonist.
- Metabolized primarily through CYP1A2 (major), and to a lesser extent CYP2C9 and CYP3A4; t ½: 1–2.6 hours.
- Avoid concomitant use with CNS depressants (additive effects). Exercise caution in patients taking potent CYP1A2 inhibitors (eg, fluvoxamine), which could increase ramelteon's effects.

CLINICAL PEARLS:
- Because ramelteon's mechanism of action relates to melatonin receptors and regulation of circadian rhythms, it does not cause patients to "feel" sedated. Often patients say that it doesn't start working for several days—however, clinical trials have shown efficacy from the first night of use. It's good to warn patients and families about this ahead of time, or they may conclude it's ineffective after a single night and stop using it.
- No evidence of abuse potential or physical dependence.
- Hormonal alterations occur very rarely and usually with high-dose (16 mg in one study) and longer-term use (six to 12 months). If unexplained amenorrhea, galactorrhea, decreased libido, or fertility problems occur, consider evaluating the patient's prolactin or testosterone levels.

FUN FACT:
Another melatonin agonist, agomelatine, has been studied as an antidepressant, partly because circadian rhythms are disrupted in depression. It is approved overseas, but the manufacturer scrapped its development in the US.

Complementary Treatments

Complementary treatments are popular among patients and their parents, but they are a mixed bag: Some are useful and safe, while others can be hazardous. Contrary to common assumptions, "natural" doesn't equal safe. With this in mind, it is important to always ask patients and families about all the products that they are using. The fact sheets in this section detail potential uses of some of these agents in child psychiatry. Few of these treatments are FDA approved for use in adults, and none are FDA approved for use in children. Clinicians need to use their best judgment and ensure that there is clear informed consent covering potential risks, benefits, and unknowns when talking with patients and families about these treatments.

If you are interested in complementary treatments (also known as natural and alternative medicine, or CAM), you will likely recommend various strategies other than the products we cover in this section. These would include exercise (helpful for depression and for preventing cognitive impairment), light therapy (for seasonal affective disorder), massage, meditation, and other modalities. CAM is often used alongside ongoing medication treatment, or it can be used alone. Be careful to consider interactions, such as use of multiple serotonergic agents.

We have included fact sheets on those natural products that have been shown to be effective via standard randomized controlled trials. Some natural products not included here might be effective but have not been adequately tested vs placebo.

Because most of these products are not regulated by the FDA, there are quality control issues. The amounts of active constituents can vary not only from brand to brand, but also from batch to batch, and some products may be adulterated with other herbs, chemicals, drugs, or toxins. Some people feel "pharmaceutical grade" (99% pure) products are better. We recommend that patients stick to well-known brands sold by trusted retailers, ideally with a label that specifies certification by organizations such as U.S. Pharmacopeia (USP), NSF International, or ConsumerLab.com. Seals of approval from these organizations don't guarantee therapeutic efficacy or safety, and they don't mean that every batch is tested, but they do indicate that the product contains the amount of the ingredient listed on the label and isn't contaminated with toxins or bacteria. Manufacturers must pay for the testing and certification; hence only a small fraction of supplements carry these seals.

For additional information, you may also find these resources helpful:

- NIH National Center for Complementary and Integrative Health: www.nccih.nih.gov/health/herbsataglance
- National Library of Medicine: www.medlineplus.gov/druginfo/herb_All.html
- Natural Medicines Comprehensive Database (requires subscription): https://naturaldatabase.therapeuticresearch.com
- Consumer Lab (requires subscription): www.consumerlab.com

COMMONLY USED COMPLEMENTARY TREATMENTS

The complementary treatments that clinicians may recommend most frequently are omega-3 fatty acids for people on antipsychotics, melatonin for sleep, and L-methylfolate for people with proven or suspected methylenetetrahydrofolate reductase (MTHFR) deficiency.

- **Omega-3 fatty acids:** Omega-3s have some limited research that suggests they may reduce relapse risk in bipolar disorder, may be beneficial in depression or ADHD, and may reduce the risk of tardive dyskinesia in children and adolescents who are on antipsychotics. A recent AHRQ comparative effectiveness review of a number of studies concluded that omega-3 supplementation as monotherapy or as augmentation was ineffective for ADHD in kids.

- **Melatonin:** Melatonin is often helpful for sleep but can cause rebound wakefulness during the night, create vivid dreams, and produce rebound insomnia when discontinued. Early reports of seizures have not been borne out, nor have concerns about melatonin causing hormonal problems. As always, use the minimum effective dose, usually 0.3–3 mg in children, perhaps up to 5 mg.

- **L-methylfolate:** L-methylfolate has been medicalized by the marketing of a prescription form and the growing popularity of MTHFR genetic testing. Although the evidence base for this practice is lackluster, the marketing has been effective. We often test for MTHFR, particularly in depressed children and teens who are not responding to antidepressant treatment. Occasionally there are clear results showing enzymatic deficiency and apparent improvement with supplementation.

LESS COMMON BUT NOTABLE TREATMENTS

- **D-cycloserine:** Early studies indicated that the amino acid D-cycloserine could boost the effectiveness of cognitive behavioral therapy when administered prior to therapy sessions, especially for OCD. More recent negative studies have tempered that enthusiasm.

- **Ginkgo biloba:** Ginkgo biloba is potentially helpful for symptoms of ADHD. We will often use it as a way to ease an understandably cautious family into more effective treatment, such as a stimulant. Ginkgo is generally considered to be safe; however, there are reports of a low but notable risk of stroke, which may have relevance for children or adolescents with medical conditions.

- **Intravenous immunoglobulin (IVIG):** IVIG is also frequently used with children with developmental challenges; in particular, it is thought by some to be helpful for ill-defined immunological dyscrasias associated with autism. Reports of positive effects in non-controlled settings are, in our view, rendered moot by the risk of giving people pooled blood products. Nevertheless, IVIG is FDA approved and prescribed in other medical conditions such as primary immunodeficiency syndromes and leukemia, so it may make sense in certain circumstances if a child has such a comorbid condition.

- **Lavender:** This is another up-and-coming supplement, with adult studies supporting the use of lavender for anxiety. Lavender-flavored burps aside, it is well tolerated except for the possibility of gynecomastia due to estrogenic effects (you'll want to avoid trying lavender in pre-pubescent kids).

- **Low-dose naltrexone (LDN):** LDN is becoming popular as well. Doses typically used are on the order of 0.06 mg/kg/day, or about 2–4 mg/day in most kids. Since naltrexone is only available in 50 mg tablets, families are relying on compounding pharmacies to prepare these ultra-low doses. LDN may be helpful for anxiety and agitation, particularly in people with autism. It has also been used for fibromyalgia, fatigue, and dissociation. While liver function testing is recommended when prescribing naltrexone for substance use treatment (usual dose 25–50 mg daily), the risks of LDN are probably minimal. Efficacy data to support its uses are also minimal at best.

- **Magnesium:** While there is some risk associated with overuse of magnesium, there are fairly consistent reports of reduced anxiety when using magnesium supplementation in children, adolescents, and adults.

- **Methyl B12 injections for autism:** These are among the most common of the "biomedical" treatments in the autism world, and as usual, the research is mixed except for the open-label cases where families report that the injections are helpful. This is probably harmless, though weekly injections can traumatize susceptible children, and injection site complications are possible.

- **N-acetylcysteine (NAC):** An amino acid, NAC may help anxiety, skin picking, obsessive-compulsive symptoms, and cannabis use disorder with no ill effects.

- **Oxytocin:** Oxytocin enjoys wide popularity as well, currently in the form of a nasal spray used twice a day at doses of 10–40 mcg. Research is mixed for improved social function in adults with autism and negligible for children. There is a theoretical concern that oxytocin might lead a vulnerable child to attach to any stranger; however, this has not been borne out.

- **S-adenosyl-L-methionine (SAMe) and St. John's wort:** SAMe and St. John's wort are widely touted to help mild to moderate depression in adults, presumably via serotonergic mechanisms similar to SSRIs. St. John's wort is routinely used in Europe. However, as with most supplements available in the US, the dosage is variable due to poor oversight of the industry and high pill-to-pill variability. We recommend caution in children due to risks of serotonergic syndrome, particularly in combination with SSRIs or SNRIs, and perhaps triptan medications used for migraine.

- **Saffron (*Crocus sativus*):** The plant that produces saffron, one of the most expensive spices and known for its bright pigment, has been touted to have benefits in depression, cardiovascular health, and erectile dysfunction. While very few high-quality studies exist, saffron has also most recently been purported to help patients with ADHD. This is based on a small pilot study of 50 children (ages 6–17 years) who completed a six-week randomized double-blind study. The half who received 20–30 mg/day of methylphenidate showed similar reduction in ADHD symptoms as the half who received saffron. Unfortunately, this was a small, short-duration study with no placebo arm. Saffron may be an option for families reluctant to try stimulants, but we are keeping an eye out for further studies.

- **Vitamin A:** Often among the mega-vitamin treatments touted for children with developmental and learning challenges, vitamin A is also toxic in high doses: 2000 IU (600 mcg) for infants and young children ages 0–3, 3000 IU (900 mcg) for ages 4–8, 5667 IU (1700 mcg) for ages 9–13, and 9333 IU (2300 mcg) for ages 14–18.

- **Vitamin D:** Reports of population-wide vitamin D deficiency and its possible association with depression and other health conditions are fueling a surge of supplementation. Vitamin D levels (25-OH vitamin D) seem to be the lab test du jour. Should we all be testing for vitamin D in children and teens? Perhaps, especially since we typically advise parents to be sure children are using sunscreen—its use lowers the risk for melanoma but also limits the natural production of vitamin D. Note that there are potential dangers in over-supplementation (greater than 5000 IU per day of vitamin D3 in adults), which can create osteoporosis secondary to hypercalcemia, renal toxicity, and hepatotoxicity.

TREATMENTS THAT ARE NOT RECOMMENDED

- **Cannabinoids:** Cannabidiol (CBD) is a component of marijuana that does not produce a high and is believed by some to help depression and schizophrenia. Safety and efficacy studies, however, are limited to two good studies demonstrating efficacy in treating intractable seizures. Tetrahydrocannabinol (THC), the psychoactive component of marijuana used recreationally, doubles psychosis risk and reduces motivation, adding to concerns about CBD since some CBD products may contain trace amounts (or potentially more) of THC. Illegal by federal law, clinicians need to weigh whether to recuse themselves from care or even contact protective services if they learn that a patient is using or being given cannabinoids. Consultation and documentation may be more critical in this scenario.

Several agents that are purported to be beneficial for psychiatric symptoms but have no evidence to support their use include secretin, colloidal silver, and pycnogenol. We do not recommend their use.

- **Secretin:** Secretin is a gastrointestinal hormone that has been used experimentally for autism. The studies have been negative, and there are significant potential hazards. For example, one secretin infusion–related death was reported a number of years ago.

- **Colloidal silver:** This is sometimes used to treat autism. However, there are no controlled efficacy studies. Side effects include permanent graying of skin.

- **Pycnogenol:** Pycnogenol is an alleged antioxidant extracted from grape seeds and pine tree bark. It has been reportedly used for autism, but no legitimate research has been published, and the cost of the treatment is high.

TABLE 10: Complementary Treatments

Name (Brand name, if applicable)	Commonly Available Strengths (mg)	Reported Uses in Psychiatry	Usual Pediatric Dosage Range (starting–max) (mg)
Lavender essential oil (Silexan, CalmAid)	80, 500	Generalized anxiety disorder, irritability in autism	80 QHS
L-methylfolate (Deplin and others)	0.4, 0.8, 1, 3, 5, 7.5, 15	Depression (adjunct)	15
Magnesium	100, 250, 400, 500	Anxiety, ADHD, insomnia	65–350
Melatonin	0.5, 1, 2.5, 3, 5, 10	Insomnia, irritability in autism	0.3–5
N-acetylcysteine	500, 600, 750, 1000	OCD, trichotillomania, nail biting, skin picking, cannabis use disorder	1200–2400
Omega-3 fatty acids (fish oil)	500, 1000, 1200	Depression (unipolar, bipolar, and ADHD, albeit evidence not supportive for ADHD), irritability in autism	500–2000
S-adenosyl-L-methionine (SAMe)	100, 200, 400	Depression	800 BID
Saffron	28, 30, 50, 60	ADHD, depression, anxiety	20–30
St. John's wort	100, 300, 450	Depression	300 TID
Vitamin D	1000 IU, 2000 IU, 5000 IU, 10,000 IU (as D3)	Depression	1000–2500 IU

LAVENDER ESSENTIAL OIL (CalmAid, Silexan) Fact Sheet [G]

BOTTOM LINE:
Lavender essential oil is a reasonable option in patients who have not responded to FDA-approved treatments for generalized anxiety disorder (GAD) or in patients and families who request a natural alternative. Given the potential risk for hormonal disruption, it should be used with caution in males and younger females.

PEDIATRIC AND ADULT FDA INDICATIONS:
None.

OFF-LABEL USES:
None.

DOSAGE FORMS:
Softgels (CalmAid): 80 mg, 500 mg.

PEDIATRIC DOSAGE GUIDANCE:
- No guidance for pediatric dosing.
- Start and continue 80 mg QHS. May consider 500 mg for adult-sized patients.

MONITORING: No routine monitoring recommended unless clinical picture warrants.

COST: $

SIDE EFFECTS:
- Most common: Lavender-flavored burping; well tolerated in most.
- Serious but rare: Weak estrogenic properties may contribute to rare cases of breast development in adolescents (avoid in those under 12), palpitations at higher doses.

MECHANISM, PHARMACOKINETICS, AND DRUG INTERACTIONS:
- Several mechanisms proposed, but most relevant may be serotonin-1A agonism.
- Drug metabolism pathway unclear; t ½: 9 hours.
- Drug interactions: Limited information, though studies thus far show no inhibition or induction of P450 enzymes by Silexan.

CLINICAL PEARLS:
- Silexan is a proprietary blend of linalool and linalyl acetate, along with over 100 compounds from the lavender plant.
- In a large randomized, double-blind controlled study in adults, Silexan 80 mg and 160 mg both beat out paroxetine 20 mg/day and placebo on the Hamilton Anxiety Rating Scale with a large effect size of 0.87. Silexan also performed best on secondary outcome measures such as depression, sleep quality, and quality of life.
- One smaller study found Silexan 80 mg/day was comparable to lorazepam 0.5 mg/day in adult patients with GAD.
- Benefits are typically seen after two weeks and continue to build over three months.
- While Silexan is not sedating, patients report improved sleep quality, likely secondary to its anxiolytic effect.
- A formulation containing 500 mg of dried lavender is also available. This has been studied (taken BID) in postmenopausal women for anxiety.

FUN FACT:
Silexan is regulated as a prescription and licensed for anxiety in 14 countries. In the US, it is available over the counter as CalmAid, through Schwabe's "Nature's Way" line.

L-METHYLFOLATE (Deplin) Fact Sheet [G]

BOTTOM LINE:
Though the data are not robust, folate supplementation *might* be effective for some kids with depression, but we recommend that patients try the cheap stuff (folic acid) before springing for Deplin (L-methylfolate).

PEDIATRIC AND ADULT FDA INDICATIONS:
None.

OFF-LABEL USES:
Adjunctive treatment for depression (considered a "medical food product" by the FDA, not an FDA-approved drug product, although available as prescription only).

DOSAGE FORMS:
- **Capsules (Deplin):** 7.5 mg, 15 mg.
- **Tablets and capsules (various other L-methylfolate products):** 0.4 mg, 0.8 mg, 1 mg, 3 mg, 5 mg.

PEDIATRIC DOSAGE GUIDANCE:
- No guidance for pediatric dosing.
- Adult dosing for depression (Deplin only): Start 7.5 mg QD; target and max dose 15 mg/day.

COST: [G]: $$; Deplin: $$$

SIDE EFFECTS:
- Most common: Not well known; likely well tolerated.
- Serious but rare: Folic acid supplementation may mask symptoms of vitamin B12 deficiency (administration of folic acid may reverse the hematological signs of B12 deficiency, including megaloblastic anemia, while not addressing neurological manifestations). L-methylfolate may be less likely than folic acid to mask B12 deficiency, though the possibility should be considered.

MECHANISM, PHARMACOKINETICS, AND DRUG INTERACTIONS:
- May enhance synthesis of monoamine neurotransmitters.
- No typical drug metabolism pathway as it is naturally stored and used by body; t ½: 3 hours.
- Drug interactions generally unlikely, although L-methylfolate may decrease anticonvulsant levels (including carbamazepine, valproic acid). Drugs that lower folate, such as anticonvulsants (including carbamazepine, valproic acid, lamotrigine), may necessitate higher doses of L-methylfolate.

EVIDENCE AND CLINICAL PEARLS:
- A few small studies in adults over the years have shown that both folate (over the counter) and L-methylfolate may be somewhat helpful as adjunctive agents in the treatment of depression, particularly in those with low baseline folate levels. No studies in pediatric patients.
- Clinicians tend to order genetic testing for MTHFR when a person's symptoms are not improving or a family member has been found to have this problem, although the evidence for the actual clinical relevance of this testing is lacking.
- Dietary folic acid is normally transformed to L-methylfolate by the enzyme MTHFR, and L-methylfolate is necessary for the synthesis of monoamines (serotonin, norepinephrine, dopamine). The marketing pitch for prescribing Deplin is that in about 50% of the population, genetic variations impair the function of MTHFR, leading to low levels of methylfolate. A recent review of the data on one of these genetic polymorphisms (called C677T) found that overall, it did not put people at any higher risk of depression—in fact, schizophrenia was more common.

FUN FACT:
"Medical foods" are foods that are specially formulated and intended for the dietary management of a disease that has distinctive nutritional needs that cannot be met by normal diet alone. These include total parenteral nutrition as well as nasogastric tube feeds and oral rehydration products. Depression has no accepted distinctive nutritional needs.

MAGNESIUM Fact Sheet [G]

BOTTOM LINE:
Magnesium supplementation may improve symptoms of ADHD or anxiety in children with a deficiency, but supporting or convincing evidence is lacking.

PEDIATRIC AND ADULT FDA INDICATIONS:
None.

OFF-LABEL USES:
Anxiety; ADHD; insomnia.

DOSAGE FORMS:
Capsules, tablets, softgels, chewables, oral liquid: 100 mg, 250 mg, 400 mg, 500 mg.

PEDIATRIC DOSAGE GUIDANCE:
- Anxiety: Max 65 mg/day for kids 1–3 years; max 110 mg/day for kids 4–8 years; max 350 mg/day for kids >8 years.
- ADHD: Magnesium aspartates and lactates 6 mg/kg/day.

COST: $

SIDE EFFECTS:
- Most common: Well tolerated, although higher doses may cause loose stools and diarrhea.
- Serious but rare: Excessive intake can lead to symptomatic hypermagnesemia, which presents as hypotension, nausea, vomiting, and bradycardia.

MECHANISM, PHARMACOKINETICS, AND DRUG INTERACTIONS:
- Essential mineral used in the human body, as a cofactor.
- Excreted in urine; t ½: unknown.
- Drug interactions generally unlikely.

EVIDENCE AND CLINICAL PEARLS:
- An overview of 18 studies in adults suggested magnesium had a beneficial effect on subjective anxiety; however, they were all poor-quality studies, and the review recommended better controlled trials.
- Magnesium supplements are formulated as various salts (citrate, chloride, gluconate, aspartate, oxide, pidolate, and orotate) or combined with other ingredients (eg, multivitamin).
- Used most often to prevent or treat deficiency or as a laxative. It is sometimes used for pregnancy-induced leg cramps or restless legs syndrome.
- In kids, it may be used for treating anxiety. Magnesium is frequently mentioned in treatment of anxiety in autism; however, research beyond case reports is lacking.
- Although the Natural Medicines database deems magnesium "insufficient reliable evidence to rate," one study suggests that elemental magnesium 300 mg/day (adults, mostly women) combined with hawthorn and California poppy (not available in the US) may be useful in the treatment of mild to moderate anxiety.
- Also considered "insufficient reliable evidence to rate" is magnesium's role in children with ADHD. Preliminary data (no randomized placebo-controlled trials) suggest supplementation may improve hyperactivity in children with ADHD who have low magnesium levels.
- Several studies in older adults have shown benefits of magnesium for insomnia. The studies were of low quality, however.

FUN FACT:
In 1618, a farmer in Epsom, England had cows who were refusing to drink from a local well. It turned out the water had a bitter taste but healed scratches and rashes. Thus was the birth of the magnesium compound: epsom salts (MgSO4-7H2O).

MELATONIN Fact Sheet [G]

BOTTOM LINE:
Short-term melatonin treatment appears to have only a modest effect size in kids with insomnia. It modestly reduces the time it takes to fall asleep (about 12 minutes) and does not appear to significantly improve overall sleep time. However, some patients and parents report minor improvement in subjective feelings of sleep quality.

PEDIATRIC AND ADULT FDA INDICATIONS:
None.

OFF-LABEL USES:
Insomnia; jet lag; shift-work sleep disorder; daytime irritability with autism.

DOSAGE FORMS:
Supplied over the counter in various forms, including liquid, tablet, capsule, sublingual, and time-release formulations; usually in 0.5 mg, 1 mg, 2.5 mg, 3 mg, 5 mg, and 10 mg.

PEDIATRIC DOSAGE GUIDANCE:
- Doses studied vary from 0.3 mg to 5 mg, and up to 5–10 mg for children with special needs, given anywhere from 30 minutes to three hours before bedtime.
- For very young children, use 0.3–1 mg. For school-aged children, use 2.5–5 mg. Some older kids and adolescents, especially autistic kids, may need up to 5–10 mg nightly.
- Insomnia (adults): 0.5–20 mg in early evening. Emerging data suggest lower doses are effective; start low (0.5–1 mg) and gradually increase to desired effect ("normal" melatonin levels vary widely among individuals, and same dose can induce different levels depending on age or health).
- For jet lag, 1–3 mg on day of departure at a time that corresponds to the anticipated bedtime at arrival destination, followed by 1–3 mg at bedtime for next three to five days.
- For delayed sleep phase syndrome, 300–500 mcg given four hours before bedtime for about three weeks, until bedtime is adjusted to desired earlier time.

COST: $

SIDE EFFECTS:
- Most common: Generally well tolerated in the short term. Only rare and mild side effects. Drowsiness, headaches, and dizziness most common but at similar rates to placebo; next-day grogginess or irritability (higher doses); vivid dreams or nightmares (higher doses).
- Serious but rare: No serious side effects reported; however, long-term human studies have not been conducted.

MECHANISM, PHARMACOKINETICS, AND DRUG INTERACTIONS:
- Melatonin receptor agonist.
- Metabolized primarily through CYP1A2, may inhibit CYP1A2; t ½: 35–50 minutes.
- Some suggest melatonin may reduce glucose tolerance and insulin sensitivity and may ↑ efficacy of calcium channel blockers for blood pressure.

EVIDENCE AND CLINICAL PEARLS:
- Melatonin is secreted from the pineal gland in a 24-hour circadian rhythm. It rises at sunset and peaks in the middle of the night, regulating the normal sleep/wake cycle.
- Good evidence and safety database in kids, much of it in autistic kids or kids with ADHD, and considered a first-line agent in many when pharmacologic intervention is indicated. Studied in kids as young as 3 years.
- A Dutch study followed kids taking melatonin for a mean of 3.1 years and found no significant long-term effects, including pubertal development.

FUN FACT:
Foods containing melatonin include cherries, bananas, grapes, rice, cereals, herbs, olive oil, wine, and beer.

Complementary Treatments

N-ACETYLCYSTEINE (NAC) Fact Sheet [G]

BOTTOM LINE:
Efficacy of NAC in a wide range of psychiatric disorders has been investigated. For now, it is best reserved as an add-on for kids only partially responding to SSRIs in OCD or the other repetitive behaviors involving hair, nails, and skin.

PEDIATRIC AND ADULT FDA INDICATIONS:
None.

OFF-LABEL USES:
OCD; trichotillomania; nail biting; skin picking; cannabis use disorder; irritability with autism.

DOSAGE FORMS:
Capsules: 500 mg, 600 mg, 750 mg, 1000 mg.

PEDIATRIC DOSAGE GUIDANCE:
- Minimal dosing guidance in pediatric patients.
- NAC doses studied have ranged from 600 mg to 6000 mg/day with majority of the studies using 1200–2400 mg/day. Divide dose BID to minimize GI side effects.

COST: $

SIDE EFFECTS:
- Most common: Usually well tolerated with nausea/vomiting, diarrhea, cramping, flatulence being most common side effects. GI symptoms usually diminish after a few weeks.
- Serious but rare: May exacerbate asthma.

MECHANISM, PHARMACOKINETICS, AND DRUG INTERACTIONS:
- NAC is derived from the amino acid cysteine, a precursor of a key brain antioxidant, glutathione. It works as a glutamate modulator, which may have effects on oxidative stress, mitochondrial dysfunction, inflammatory mediators, neurotransmission, and neural plasticity.
- Metabolized extensively by liver with minimal P450 involvement; t ½: 6 hours.
- No known drug interactions; not likely an issue for the majority of patients.

EVIDENCE AND CLINICAL PEARLS:
- Amino acid derivate with antioxidant properties.
- NAC is most recognized for its use as a treatment for acetaminophen overdose.
- Although NAC has been studied in autism, Alzheimer's, cocaine and cannabis addiction, bipolar disorder, depression, trichotillomania, nail biting, skin picking, OCD, and schizophrenia, the results are generally mixed. Best data are in patients with OCD, trichotillomania, nail biting, and skin picking (including Prader-Willi syndrome).
- Majority of data are in adults. Data in kids are limited to case reports and a small (n = 34) randomized clinical trial in kids with OCD, which showed statistically significant improvement in the group that had NAC added to citalopram compared to placebo and citalopram.

FUN FACT:
Many of the published studies have come from an individual Australian researcher who holds a patent on a particular formulation of NAC, raising the issue of bias or a potential conflict of interest.

OMEGA-3 FATTY ACIDS (Fish Oil) Fact Sheet [G]

BOTTOM LINE:
Based on the limited data available, the best use of omega-3 fatty acids (particularly 1–2 g with at least 60% EPA) is as an adjunct in the treatment of unipolar and bipolar depression.

PEDIATRIC FDA INDICATIONS:
None.

ADULT FDA INDICATIONS:
High triglycerides (as Lovaza); no FDA indications in psychiatry.

OFF-LABEL USES:
Unipolar and bipolar depression; prevention of tardive dyskinesia; maintenance of mood stability for bipolar disorder.

DOSAGE FORMS:
- Supplied over the counter in various dosages and formulations; 500 mg, 1000 mg, and 1200 mg softgel capsules most common.
- By prescription only: Lovaza: 1000 mg softgel capsules (GSK). Dosage on label usually reflects fish oil dosage, which is not the same as omega-3 fatty acid dosage (eg, 1000 mg fish oil in some brands may provide 300 mg of omega-3 fatty acids, including EPA and DHA). Dosing recommendations are based on mg of fish oil.

PEDIATRIC DOSAGE GUIDANCE:
Effective dose unclear, but studies in children have used 300 mg–1.5 g QD. For depression, start 500 mg/day, increase as tolerated (target dose 1–2 g/day); doses >2–3 g/day should be used cautiously. Dividing dose BID–TID helps with side effect tolerability. For ADHD, typical dosages are 1200–1500 mg daily with EPA higher than DHA.

COST: $

SIDE EFFECTS:
- Most common: Well tolerated up to 4 g/day. Nausea, loose stools, fishy aftertaste.
- Serious but rare: Caution in those who are allergic to seafood. Increased risk of bleeding, particularly at higher doses.

MECHANISM, PHARMACOKINETICS, AND DRUG INTERACTIONS:
- Exact mechanism unknown, but may improve cell membrane fluidity and membrane function, change neurotransmitter binding, and promote anti-inflammatory effects.
- Metabolism is hepatic, primarily through CYP450; t ½: unknown.
- For most patients, drug interactions not likely an issue; however, may prolong bleeding time. Fish oils may lower blood pressure and have additive effects when used with antihypertensives.

EVIDENCE AND CLINICAL PEARLS:
- A meta-analysis of 10 trials in 699 children with ADHD treated with omega-3 showed modest efficacy. However, a recent AHRQ comparative effectiveness review concluded omega-3 supplementation is not effective for ADHD based on review of a number of studies of kids with ADHD. While evidence is lacking, omega-3 is used at times for ADHD, and so we have included it here.
- Fish oils contain eicosapentaenoic acid (EPA) and docosahexaenoic acid (DHA); both are omega-3 fatty acids (which form the lipid bilayers of cell membranes). Although the body can synthesize these fats from alpha-linolenic acid (ALA), this is believed to be inefficient in many people.
- Mercury accumulates in fish meat more than in fish oil, which might explain the lack of detectable mercury in most fish oil supplements. Also, questions about increased bleeding risk have not been borne out in research studies.
- Look for formulations with higher EPA than DHA content, typically at least a 1.5 to 1 ratio (eg, 600 mg EPA to 400 mg DHA).
- Omega-3 fatty acids appear helpful as augmentation in unipolar depression in some individual studies, but several meta-analyses have not been able to show robust benefit.

FUN FACT:
Inuit people have been reported to ingest up to 16 g/day (via fish) with no dangerous side effects.

Complementary Treatments

S-ADENOSYL-L-METHIONINE (SAMe) Fact Sheet [G]

BOTTOM LINE:
Very minimal data in pediatric patients. Consider using it for those patients with mild to moderate depression who are interested in using alternative therapies, or as an augmentation strategy in partial responders.

PEDIATRIC AND ADULT FDA INDICATIONS:
None.

OFF-LABEL USES:
Depression; osteoarthritis; cirrhosis and fatty liver disease.

DOSAGE FORMS:
Supplied over the counter most often as 100 mg, 200 mg, 400 mg tablets, usually enteric-coated.

PEDIATRIC DOSAGE GUIDANCE:
- No pediatric dosage guidance.
- Effective dose is variable, but most adult antidepressant studies have used doses of about 400–1600 mg/day (1600 mg/day most common), usually divided BID.

COST: $

SIDE EFFECTS:
- Most common: Well tolerated. Higher doses may result in flatulence, nausea, vomiting, diarrhea, constipation, dry mouth, headache, mild insomnia, anorexia, sweating, dizziness, and nervousness. Anxiety and tiredness have occurred in people with depression, and hypomania has occurred in people with bipolar disorder.
- Serious but rare: Theoretical concern of elevated homocysteine since SAMe is converted to this during normal metabolism. No reports to date, but some recommend taking folate and vitamin B supplements anyway.

MECHANISM, PHARMACOKINETICS, AND DRUG INTERACTIONS:
- Methyl group donor that may increase synthesis of neurotransmitters, increase responsiveness of neurotransmitter receptors, and increase fluidity of cell membranes through the production of phospholipids.
- Metabolism similar to endogenous SAMe (transmethylation, trans-sulphuration, and amino-propylation); t ½: 100 minutes.
- No drug interactions reported. Theoretically, serotonin syndrome possible, but risk is likely minimal.

EVIDENCE AND CLINICAL PEARLS:
- Only one small study (n = 3) in pediatric depression showed SAMe 400–1200 mg/day improved symptoms and was well tolerated.
- SAMe is difficult to formulate as a stable oral salt, and the FDA halted trials of an investigational prescription product in 1993 due to concerns about tablet dissolution; concerns have been raised that some supplements may also have these problems.

FUN FACTS:
SAMe has been available as a dietary supplement in the US since 1999, but it has been used as a prescription drug in Italy since 1979, in Spain since 1985, and in Germany since 1989. Patients in trials of SAMe for depression noted improvement in their arthritis symptoms, suggesting another possible use.

SAFFRON Fact Sheet [G]

BOTTOM LINE:
A very limited number of studies (mostly in adults) have shown promise for saffron in ADHD, depression, and anxiety. It's likely safe to use, so you may consider it for patients with milder symptoms or who are reluctant to take medications.

PEDIATRIC AND ADULT FDA INDICATIONS:
None.

OFF-LABEL USES:
Depression; anxiety; ADHD.

DOSAGE FORMS:
Capsules: 15 mg, 28 mg, 30 mg, 50 mg, 60 mg.

PEDIATRIC DOSAGE GUIDANCE:
- No guidance for pediatric dosing. One study in ADHD used 20–30 mg/day in kids.
- Start and continue 20 mg/day for kids <30 kg and 30 mg/day for >30 kg.

MONITORING: No routine monitoring recommended unless clinical picture warrants.

COST: $

SIDE EFFECTS:
- Most common: Agitation possible; well tolerated in most.
- Serious but rare: Unknown.

MECHANISM, PHARMACOKINETICS, AND DRUG INTERACTIONS:
- Several mechanisms proposed, but most relevant may be related to anti-inflammatory and antioxidant properties.
- Drug metabolism pathway unclear; t ½: 6–7.5 hours.
- Drug interactions: Limited information, unknown.

CLINICAL PEARLS:
- Saffron contains more than 150 chemicals, but the two most biologically active are thought to be crocin and crocetin.
- In Chinese medicine, saffron is used for the treatment of depression, irregular menstruation, postpartum thrombosis, and bruises.
- Two small controlled studies in adults (one in combination with curcumin) demonstrated greater efficacy with saffron than placebo in patients with depression. Saffron has also been shown to be equally effective as antidepressants (citalopram, fluoxetine, imipramine) in mild to moderate adult depression.
- One adult study showed saffron 25 mg/day to be more effective than diazepam 5 mg/day in reducing anxiety.
- A randomized controlled pilot study of 50 children (6–17 years) with ADHD showed no difference in efficacy (per Teacher and Parent Attention-Deficit/Hyperactivity Disorder Rating Scale-IV) between saffron 20–30 mg/day and methylphenidate 20–30 mg/day. There was no placebo arm, and the study duration was only six weeks, so larger studies with longer treatment duration will be helpful to determine saffron's role in ADHD.

FUN FACT:
Saffron, the dried red stigma of the perennial herb *Crocus sativus L.*, is the most expensive spice in the world.

Complementary Treatments

ST. JOHN'S WORT Fact Sheet [G]

BOTTOM LINE:
St. John's wort can be considered an option for short-term treatment of mild depression in adults, but for kids the evidence is weaker.

PEDIATRIC AND ADULT FDA INDICATIONS:
None.

OFF-LABEL USES:
Depression.

DOSAGE FORMS:
Supplied over the counter most commonly as 100 mg, 300 mg, 450 mg tablets and capsules.

PEDIATRIC DOSAGE GUIDANCE:
- For mild to moderate depression, most clinical trials have used St. John's wort extract containing 0.3% hypericin and/or 3% hyperforin. Most common dose is 300 mg TID; doses of 1200 mg QD have also been used.
- Some studies have used a 0.2% hypericin extract dosed at 250 mg BID.
- A St. John's wort extract standardized to 5% hyperforin and dosed at 300 mg TID has also been used.

COST: $

SIDE EFFECTS:
- Most common: Well tolerated at recommended doses. Insomnia (decrease dose or take in morning), vivid dreams, restlessness, anxiety, agitation, irritability, gastrointestinal discomfort, diarrhea, fatigue, dry mouth, dizziness, and headache reported. Sexual dysfunction may occur, but less often than with SSRIs.
- Serious but rare: Risk of severe phototoxic skin reactions and photosensitivity at high doses (2–4 g/day).

MECHANISM, PHARMACOKINETICS, AND DRUG INTERACTIONS:
- Thought to exert antidepressant effects by modulating effects of monoamines, and may inhibit reuptake of these neurotransmitters.
- Metabolized primarily through the liver; t ½: 24–48 hours.
- Avoid concomitant use with serotonergic agents: Rare cases of serotonin syndrome reported. Potent inducer of many CYP450 enzymes (3A4, 2C9, 1A2) and P-glycoprotein transporter, which results in increased metabolism and reduced plasma concentrations of a large number of drugs. St. John's wort can decrease oral contraceptive levels by 13%–15%, resulting in bleeding or unplanned pregnancy; women should use an additional or nonhormonal form of birth control.

EVIDENCE AND CLINICAL PEARLS:
- Adult studies have been mixed, but most have reported St. John's wort is more effective than placebo, likely as effective as low-dose TCAs and SSRIs in milder forms of depression.
- No quality studies in pediatric depression. One randomized trial in pediatric ADHD (n = 54) found no benefit of St. John's wort 300 mg TID over placebo.

FUN FACTS:
Although not indigenous to Australia and long considered a weed, St. John's wort is now grown as a cash crop, and Australia produces 20% of the world's supply. St. John's wort is so named because it blooms near June 24th, which is the birthday of John the Baptist. "Wort" is an old English word for plant.

VITAMIN D Fact Sheet [G]

BOTTOM LINE:
Vitamin D supplementation may be beneficial in adults with depression, but there is only minimal evidence in pediatric patients with mania. Reserve its use for those who have insufficiency, and have your patients take 1000–2000 IU daily.

PEDIATRIC AND ADULT FDA INDICATIONS:
None.

OFF-LABEL USES:
Depression.

DOSAGE FORMS:
Supplied over the counter as vitamin D2 and D3, as tablets, capsules, and softgels in "international units" (IU) dosing. We recommend D3: 1000 IU, 2000 IU, 5000 IU.

PEDIATRIC DOSAGE GUIDANCE:
Dosing guidelines vary. For depression, use 1000–2500 IU per day.

COST: $

SIDE EFFECTS:
- Most common: Well tolerated.
- Serious but rare: Vitamin D toxicity possible but very rare. Osteoporosis with doses over 5000 IU per day, and dietary habits such as excessive consumption of carbonated beverages may exacerbate this risk.

MECHANISM, PHARMACOKINETICS, AND DRUG INTERACTIONS:
- Thought to play a role in brain plasticity, neuroimmunomodulation, and inflammation.
- Metabolized by liver and kidneys; t ½: 12–50 days (varies based on level, source, dose, obesity, race).
- No known significant interactions.

EVIDENCE AND CLINICAL PEARLS:
- Several meta-analyses have found no beneficial effects of vitamin D supplementation in adults with depression. When studies were limited to depressed patients with both vitamin D insufficiency at baseline and adequate dosing of supplementation (>800 mg/day), statistically significant benefits were seen. No studies in pediatric depression.
- One small (n = 16) open-label study of vitamin D3 2000 IU daily in kids (6–17 years) with symptoms of mania showed improvement in mood symptoms.
- Sources of vitamin D include exposure to sunlight, dietary intake, and supplements.
- It's difficult to obtain sufficient daily needs from dietary intake alone. Two types of vitamin D are obtained from dietary sources: D2 (ergocalciferol) from plant sources such as mushrooms and soy milk and D3 (cholecalciferol) from animal sources such as raw fish, mackerel, and smoked salmon. D3 is approximately three times stronger than D2.
- The majority of vitamin D is produced through conversion of 7-dehydrocholesterol via ultraviolet B, after penetration of sunlight on the skin, to vitamin D3.
- Vitamin D is metabolized in the liver to 25-hydroxyvitamin D or 25(OH)D and then in the kidneys to its active form calcitriol, or 1,25-dihydroxyvitamin D. Labs will usually report 25(OH)D level with 30–60 ng/mL as normal range, 21–29 ng/mL as insufficiency, and ≤20 ng/mL as deficiency.

FUN FACT:
A number of things affect a person's vitamin D status, including distance from the equator, community air quality, skin color, and use of sunscreen.

Complementary Treatments

Mood Stabilizers

The diagnosis of bipolar disorder in youth has shifted over time; while still largely reserved for post-pubertal adolescents, some studies, mostly in the US, encompass a larger age range, including preschool-aged children. Symptom overlap and high comorbidity with ADHD require thorough assessment, particularly with younger children who likely have ADHD alone. With changes made in the DSM-5, more children may now fall into the category of disruptive mood dysregulation disorder (DMDD) instead of the catchall diagnosis of bipolar disorder NOS. It is important to note the gravity of making a clear diagnosis prior to considering medication management, as the treatment options leave much to be desired. Functional family therapy and family psychoeducation have been demonstrated to have positive effects for prodromal bipolar symptoms and early phases of bipolar disorder.

The largest study examining the efficacy of mood stabilizers for children and adolescents is the Treatment of Early Age Mania (TEAM) study, which compared risperidone, lithium, and valproic acid in a randomized controlled trial of 279 subjects never treated with mood stabilizers. Risperidone was found to be more effective than either lithium or valproic acid in the treatment of an active manic or mixed episode. Some data support the use of lamotrigine for bipolar depression in teens; however, there remains a paucity of treatment options for bipolar depression.

Mainstay options are the classic mood stabilizers. These include lithium and anticonvulsants such as valproic acid, lamotrigine, carbamazepine, and antipsychotics.

- Lithium is effective for mania and yields a demonstrated reduction in suicidal behaviors and suicide rates when compared to placebo. Disadvantages include a number of side effects, a narrow therapeutic window, congenital risks in the first trimester, and potential longer-term harm to kidney function.
- Valproic acid is also effective for mania, but try to avoid it in patients who may become pregnant, both because it is teratogenic and because it increases the risk of polycystic ovary syndrome (PCOS).
- Lamotrigine could be considered for maintenance therapy; however, downsides include the slow titration schedule, increased risk of rash in children, and limited pediatric data.
- Carbamazepine would not be considered a first-line option, but it has a couple of open-label studies that showed improvements in depression and mania. Oxcarbazepine has even fewer data to support its use in both the adult and pediatric population.
- Second-generation antipsychotics (SGAs) are considered a first-line option for pediatric bipolar disorder. Despite serious metabolic side effects, they are favored for their ease of use and the evidence supporting their effectiveness. Lurasidone and olanzapine/fluoxetine have FDA approval for pediatric bipolar depression, while asenapine, risperidone, aripiprazole, olanzapine, and quetiapine have FDA approval for acute mania/mixed episodes. For detailed information about specific agents, refer to the Antipsychotics chapter.

STOPPING MOOD STABILIZERS

Maintenance therapy is recommended for bipolar disorder; however, there will be times that mood stabilizers need to be discontinued or cross-tapered. This includes serious side effects such as a rash with lamotrigine, renal problems with lithium, or neuroleptic malignant syndrome with SGAs. In a world where many bipolar diagnoses are broad spectrum and teens develop more prefrontal inhibitory control in early adulthood, you may be able to reduce and discontinue mood stabilizers. However, patients with more classic bipolar disorder are unlikely to do well off medication. Given the high risk of relapse, a gradual taper is recommended over a minimum of four weeks, if not longer. Continued monitoring is recommended for early signs of mood symptoms.

SIDE EFFECTS AND CLASS WARNINGS

- Class warning for suicidality: All antiepileptics include this warning based on an analysis of anticonvulsant trials for a wide range of diagnoses, which demonstrated an increased risk of suicidal thoughts or behaviors from one week through 24 weeks of treatment compared to placebo. This risk was also noted to be higher in patients with a seizure disorder.
- Black box warning of lithium toxicity, with monitoring required for lithium levels given the narrow therapeutic window. Target levels range from 0.6 to 1.2 mEq/L, although mild toxicity can also occur within the normal range. Toxicity can involve confusion, ataxia, tremors, myoclonus, fasciculations, GI symptoms, renal symptoms, and arrhythmia.
- Hypersensitivity reactions: Some antiepileptic medications, including valproic acid and lamotrigine, include a warning for DRESS (drug rash with eosinophilia and systemic symptoms)/multi-organ hypersensitivity reactions, which may be life-threatening or fatal. Symptoms may include fever, lymphadenopathy, or rash. Skin precautions are important (eg, sun protection).
- Abrupt discontinuation of anticonvulsant medications may lead to rebound seizures and should generally be avoided if possible.
- GI adverse effects are common with lithium and anticonvulsants. Fatigue and sedation, as well as cognitive side effects, can occur with these medications. Drowsy driving is a particular hazard.

Mood Stabilizers

- Metabolic side effects associated with weight gain may occur with antipsychotics and mood stabilizers, with the exception of lamotrigine and topiramate.
- Menstrual changes may occur with lithium and several anticonvulsants.

Bipolar I Treatment Algorithm for Children and Adolescents

*Denotes off label

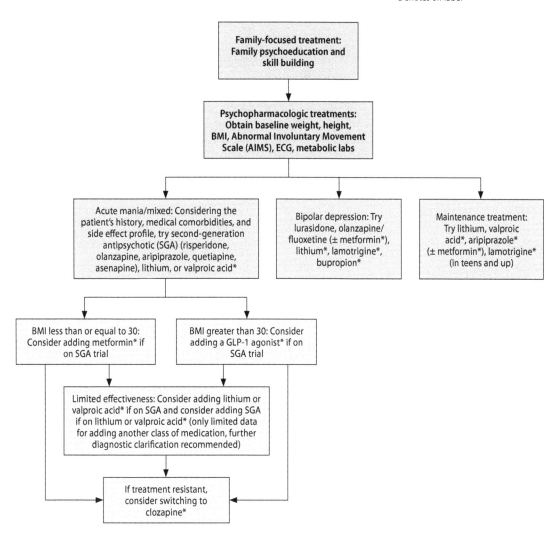

Family-focused treatment:
Family psychoeducation and skill building

↓

Psychopharmacologic treatments:
Obtain baseline weight, height, BMI, Abnormal Involuntary Movement Scale (AIMS), ECG, metabolic labs

Acute mania/mixed: Considering the patient's history, medical comorbidities, and side effect profile, try second-generation antipsychotic (SGA) (risperidone, olanzapine, aripiprazole, quetiapine, asenapine), lithium, or valproic acid*

Bipolar depression: Try lurasidone, olanzapine/fluoxetine (± metformin*), lithium*, lamotrigine*, bupropion*

Maintenance treatment: Try lithium, valproic acid*, aripiprazole* (± metformin*), lamotrigine* (in teens and up)

BMI less than or equal to 30: Consider adding metformin* if on SGA trial

BMI greater than 30: Consider adding a GLP-1 agonist* if on SGA trial

Limited effectiveness: Consider adding lithium or valproic acid* if on SGA and consider adding SGA if on lithium or valproic acid* (only limited data for adding another class of medication, further diagnostic clarification recommended)

If treatment resistant, consider switching to clozapine*

- Use non-pharmacologic approaches first when possible to help reduce use of medication
- See text and tables for specific age-related guidance
- If using antidepressants, discuss potential side effects including rare but possible increase in behavioral activation or suicidal thinking
- If using antipsychotics, check weight and labs (lipids, HbA1c, others as indicated) at baseline, 12 weeks, and yearly or sooner, AIMS at baseline and every 6 months or sooner, and consider ECG at baseline and yearly or sooner
- General guidance supports ongoing maintenance treatment; use clinical judgment if considering gradual taper or discontinuation of medications

CARLAT PUBLISHING © 2023

Mood Stabilizers

TABLE 11: Mood Stabilizers

Generic Name (Brand Name) Year FDA Approved for Bipolar Disorder or Mania [G] denotes generic availability	Relevant FDA Indication(s) (Pediatric FDA approval bolded)	Available Strengths (mg)	Usual Pediatric Dosage Range (mg)	Comments
Carbamazepine [G] (Carbatrol, Epitol, Equetro, Tegretol, Tegretol XR, Teril) 2004	Bipolar disorder (Equetro: acute mania)	CH: 100, 200 IR: 100, 200, 300, 400 ER: 100, 200, 300, 400 Oral solution: 100 mg/5 mL	200–1200	Open-label data only, but safety data in kids for seizures
Lamotrigine [G] (Lamictal, Lamictal CD, Lamictal ODT, Lamictal XR, Subvenite) 2003	Bipolar disorder (maintenance)	IR: 25, 50, 100, 150, 200 CH: 2, 5, 25 ODT: 25, 50, 100, 200 ER: 25, 50, 100, 200, 250, 300	100–400	Open-label data; caution: rash risk greater in kids
Lithium [G] (Eskalith, Lithobid) 1970	**Acute mania Bipolar maintenance (7–17 yrs)**	IR: 150, 300, 600 ER: 300, 450 Oral solution: 300 mg/5 mL	300–2400	FDA indication in kids; first-line choice
Oxcarbazepine [G] (Oxtellar XR, Trileptal) 2000[1]	Not approved for any bipolar indication	IR: 150, 300, 600 ER: 150, 300, 600 Oral suspension: 300 mg/5 mL	600–2400	No positive efficacy data to support use in kids, but safety data in kids with seizures
Valproic acid [G] (Depakene, Depakote, Depakote ER, Depakote Sprinkles) 1995	Bipolar disorder (acute mania)	IR: 250 Liquid: 250 mg/5 mL DR: 125, 250, 500 ER: 250, 500	500–2000	Open-label data only, but safety data in kids for seizures; first-line choice in acute mania but caution otherwise, particularly regarding reproductive health

CH = chewable, IR = immediate release, ER = extended release, ODT = orally disintegrating tablet, DR = delayed release

[1] Oxcarbazepine FDA approved for seizure disorder

CARBAMAZEPINE (Tegretol) Fact Sheet [G]

BOTTOM LINE:
Not a first-line treatment for bipolar disorder in kids due to limited data, side effect profile, and high likelihood of significant interactions. Used in kids for seizure disorders, so we have some basis of safety information. Equetro is FDA approved for bipolar disorder (in adults), but other cheaper formulations give similar results.

PEDIATRIC FDA INDICATIONS:
Seizure disorders.

ADULT FDA INDICATIONS:
Seizures; trigeminal neuralgia; bipolar disorder (Equetro: acute mania).

OFF-LABEL USES:
Bipolar maintenance; impulse control disorders; violence and aggression; migraine prophylaxis.

DOSAGE FORMS:
- **Chewable tablets (G):** 100 mg, 200 mg (scored).
- **Tablets (Tegretol, Epitol, [G]):** 100 mg, 200 mg, 300 mg, 400 mg (scored).
- **ER tablets (Tegretol XR, [G]):** 100 mg, 200 mg, 400 mg.
- **ER capsules (Equetro, Carbatrol, [G]):** 100 mg, 200 mg, 300 mg.
- **Oral solution (Tegretol, Teril, [G]):** 100 mg/5 mL.

PEDIATRIC DOSAGE GUIDANCE:
- Age <6 years: Start 10–20 mg/kg/day divided BID–QID, increase by 5–10 mg/kg/day in weekly intervals; max 35 mg/kg/day.
- Age 6–12 years: Start 100 mg BID, increase by 100 mg/day in weekly intervals; max 1000 mg/day in divided doses.
- Age >12 years: Start 200 mg BID and gradually ↑ by 200 mg/day in weekly intervals; max 1200 mg/day.
- Dosing is the same for IR and ER versions of carbamazepine; both are BID.

MONITORING: CBC, electrolytes (sodium), LFTs, pregnancy test, serum level, HLA-B*1502 (Asians), ECG if cardiac risk.

COST: $

SIDE EFFECTS:
- Most common: Dizziness, somnolence, nausea, headache. (ER versions may cause fewer side effects in some patients, but the evidence is not clear.)
- Serious but rare: Hematologic abnormalities including agranulocytosis, aplastic anemia, neutropenia, leukopenia, thrombocytopenia, and pancytopenia reported; hepatic complications including slight increases in hepatic enzymes, cholestatic and hepatocellular jaundice, hepatitis (and, rarely, hepatic failure), hyponatremia, SIADH; rash (5%–10%), including exfoliation, reported. Severe reactions, including toxic epidermal necrolysis and Stevens-Johnson syndrome, are rare but can be fatal.

MECHANISM, PHARMACOKINETICS, AND DRUG INTERACTIONS:
- Sodium channel blocker. Metabolized primarily through CYP3A4; t ½: 15 hours (initially 25–65 hours but induces its own metabolism over approximately two to four weeks with each dosage change and then stabilizes).
- Highly significant interactions: Potent inducer of CYP1A2, CYP2B6, CYP2C19, CYP2C8, CYP2C9, CYP3A4, P-glycoprotein; medications significantly metabolized through these pathways may become subtherapeutic; caution in patients taking strong CYP3A4 inducers or inhibitors that can affect carbamazepine levels.
- Avoid use with oral contraceptives (lowers levels/unplanned pregnancies) and clozapine (agranulocytosis).

EVIDENCE AND CLINICAL PEARLS:
- Pediatric bipolar data limited to open-label studies with only modest response rates (38%–44%).
- Therapeutic level: 4–12 mcg/mL in seizure disorders. No correlation in bipolar disorder—best dosed clinically. Check levels five days and a few weeks after changes due to induction of enzymes that affect levels.
- Avoid use if variant HLA-B*1502 allele (Asians): Risk of Stevens-Johnson syndrome/toxic epidermal necrolysis.

FUN FACT:
May cause false-positive TCA screen as its chemical structure contains the tricyclic nucleus common to TCAs.

LAMOTRIGINE (Lamictal, Subvenite) Fact Sheet [G]

BOTTOM LINE:
Not for first-line use for most kids due to limited data (open-label studies only), long titration required, and increased relative risk of rash in pediatric population.

PEDIATRIC FDA INDICATIONS:
Seizures.

ADULT FDA INDICATIONS:
Bipolar disorder (maintenance) in adults; seizures.

OFF-LABEL USES:
Bipolar depression; neuropathic pain; major depression; borderline personality disorder.

DOSAGE FORMS:
- **Tablets (Lamictal, Subvenite, [G]):** 25 mg, 50 mg, 100 mg, 150 mg, 200 mg (scored).
- **Chewable tablets (Lamictal CD, [G]):** 2 mg, 5 mg, 25 mg.
- **Orally disintegrating tablets (Lamictal ODT, [G]):** 25 mg, 50 mg, 100 mg, 200 mg.
- **ER tablets (Lamictal XR, [G]):** 25 mg, 50 mg, 100 mg, 200 mg, 250 mg, 300 mg.

PEDIATRIC DOSAGE GUIDANCE (BASED ON DOSING IN KIDS WITH SEIZURES):
- Bipolar disorder: Start 25 mg QD for two weeks, ↑ to 50 mg QD for two weeks, then 100 mg QD; max 200 mg/day.
- Patients on valproate: Start 25 mg QOD (every other day) for two weeks, ↑ to 25 mg QD for two weeks, then 50 mg QD; max 100 mg/day (VPA doubles lamotrigine levels).
- Dosing is the same with all versions of lamotrigine.

MONITORING: While some clinicians get blood levels, no specific monitoring is needed unless you are checking for compliance or toxicity.

COST: IR: $; ER: $$

SIDE EFFECTS:
- Most common: Dizziness, headache, nausea, sedation, benign rash (7%).
- Serious but rare: Rare, potentially life-threatening skin reactions (black box warning) requiring hospitalization reported, including Stevens-Johnson syndrome/toxic epidermal necrolysis; incidence higher in pediatric patients; risk increased by co-administration with valproic acid, higher-than-recommended starting doses, and exceeding recommended dose titration. Other risk factors include infections (herpes simplex, herpes zoster, HIV, hepatitis A, pneumonia), compromised immunity, and HLA-B*1502 (common in India, China, and Southeast Asia). Usually occurs before eight weeks, with isolated cases beyond eight weeks and without risk factors. Have patients take skin precautions (eg, use sunscreen; don't change detergents, soaps, or cosmetics; and avoid contact with poisonous plants). Discontinue at first sign of rash and do not reinitiate unless rash is clearly not drug related; rare cases of hemophagocytic lymphohistiocytosis (HLH) and angioedema reported. Cardiac arrhythmias (slowed ventricular conduction and widening of the QRS) in susceptible patients.

MECHANISM, PHARMACOKINETICS, AND DRUG INTERACTIONS:
- Sodium channel blocker. Metabolism primarily hepatic (non-P450); t ½: 25–33 hours (with VPA 48–70 hours; with carbamazepine 13–14 hours).
- Enzyme-inducing medications (eg, carbamazepine) and hormonal contraceptives decrease lamotrigine levels; lamotrigine may need to be increased (two-fold). Gradual increases of lamotrigine levels may occur during the inactive "pill-free" week. Lamotrigine may decrease hormonal contraceptives (estrogens more than progestins); consider alternative birth control methods. Valproic acid may double lamotrigine levels, necessitating much slower titration or dosage adjustments (as above).

EVIDENCE AND CLINICAL PEARLS:
- One open-label response: Monotherapy in pediatric bipolar disorder, 54% for manic symptoms.
- For maintenance in adult bipolar disorder; prophylaxis of depression. Not useful in acute episodes.
- If stopped/missed >5 half-lives (see above), restart with initial dosing protocol to minimize rash risk.
- FDA warning: Rare cases of HLH, a life-threatening immune reaction. Refer immediately for persistent fever (>101°F); rash; pain, tenderness, or swelling in the area of the liver; swollen lymph nodes; jaundice; unusual bleeding; and nervous system problems such as seizures, trouble walking, or visual difficulties.

FUN FACT:
The first FDA-approved drug for bipolar disorder in adults (not just acute mania) since lithium, a drug approved more than 30 years earlier (2003 for lamotrigine, 1970 for lithium).

LITHIUM (Eskalith, Lithobid) Fact Sheet [G]

BOTTOM LINE:
Although clinicians often try other medications first due to both the relative complexity of managing lithium as well as bias from the public, lithium, along with several second-generation antipsychotics, is FDA indicated and considered first line for treating pediatric bipolar disorder. Although it is not free from side effects, most common effects can be managed quite well.

PEDIATRIC FDA INDICATIONS:
Acute mania; bipolar disorder maintenance (7–17 years).

ADULT FDA INDICATIONS:
Acute mania; bipolar disorder maintenance.

OFF-LABEL USES:
Bipolar depression; treatment-resistant depression; neutropenia; vascular headache.

DOSAGE FORMS:
- **Capsules (lithium carbonate, [G]):** 150 mg, 300 mg, 600 mg.
- **Tablets (lithium carbonate, [G]):** 300 mg.
- **ER tablets: Lithobid, [G]:** 300 mg; **Eskalith CR, [G]:** 450 mg (scored).
- **Oral solution (lithium citrate, [G]):** 300 mg/5 mL.

PEDIATRIC DOSAGE GUIDANCE (DOSING SAME FOR IR AND ER VERSIONS; BOTH MAY BE BID OR QHS):
- <30 kg: Start 10 mg/kg/day divided BID–QID, increase by 5–10 mg/kg/day in weekly intervals to target dose 15–40 mg/kg/day divided TID–QID; max 60 mg/kg/day.
- >30 kg: Start 10–20 mg/kg/day divided BID–QID, increase by 10 mg/kg/day in weekly intervals to target dose 15–40 mg/kg/day divided TID–QID; max 60 mg/kg/day.
- Adolescents: Start 600–900 mg/day divided BID–TID, increase by 300 mg/day in weekly intervals to target dose 900–1200 mg/day divided TID–QID; max 2400 mg/day.

MONITORING: TSH, BUN/creatinine, CBC, basic metabolic panel, weight, pregnancy test, serum drug level, ECG if cardiac disease or older patient.

COST: $

SIDE EFFECTS:
- Most common: Nausea/diarrhea (take with meals, split dosing, switch to ER), fine tremor (lower dose or use propranolol), polyuria/excessive thirst (dose all at bedtime), memory problems, weight gain, hypothyroidism (7%–8%; nine times more common in women), acne or worsening psoriasis, benign increase in WBC.
- Serious but rare: Chronic use may result in diminished renal concentrating ability (nephrogenic diabetes insipidus); usually reverses when discontinued, or treat with hydrochlorothiazide 25–50 mg/day or amiloride 5–10 mg twice daily. Cardiac: Bradycardia, cardiac arrhythmia, flattened or inverted T waves, sinus node dysfunction may occur rarely; normal pressure hydrocephalus characterized by loss of bladder control, delirium, and ataxia (wet, wild, and wobbly). These side effects require immediate discontinuation and possibly dialysis to extract lithium from the patient.

MECHANISM, PHARMACOKINETICS, AND DRUG INTERACTIONS:
- Alters neuronal sodium transport.
- Eliminated by kidneys; t ½: 18–24 hours.
- Drugs that increase lithium levels: "**N**o **ACE** in the **H**ole" (**N**SAIDs, **ACE** inhibitors, and **H**CTZ); excess sweating can increase levels; low-sodium diet may increase lithium levels. Caffeine may decrease levels.

EVIDENCE AND CLINICAL PEARLS:
- Four open-label trials of lithium in pediatric bipolar disorder suggest efficacy; only one of these was monotherapy (with a 38% response rate). More recent double-blind studies did not show benefit over placebo in mania, yet lithium is FDA indicated for kids >7 years.
- Check lithium level, TSH/T4, BUN/Cr, CBC, BMP, electrolytes after one week of treatment, at one to two months, then every six to 12 months. Target levels for acute mania: 0.8–1.2 mEq/L; maintenance: 0.6–1.0 mEq/L; toxicity >1.5 mEq/L, but may see signs at lower levels. Levels should be drawn 12 hours after a dose; steady state generally reached after five days.
- An increase or decrease of 300 mg/day will change serum level by roughly 0.25±0.1 mEq/L.
- Dehydration: Use with caution in patients with significant fluid loss (protracted sweating, diarrhea, or prolonged fever); temporary reduction or discontinuation may be necessary.
- Shown to have anti-suicide effects in bipolar and unipolar mood disorders in adults.

FUN FACTS:
The soft drink 7-Up was originally called "Bib-Label Lithiated Lemon-Lime Soda" and contained lithium until 1950.

Mood Stabilizers

OXCARBAZEPINE (Oxtellar XR, Trileptal) Fact Sheet [G]

BOTTOM LINE:
Compared to carbamazepine, oxcarbazepine poses less concern for drug interactions and for hepatic or hematologic toxicities; it also does not require serum level monitoring. However, due to lack of efficacy data in pediatric bipolar disorder, we do not recommend its general use for that disorder. Still, some clinicians use oxcarbazepine to try to reduce irritability in a wider range of clinical circumstances. It is reserved for third-line use after lithium and valproic acid, and even after carbamazepine.

PEDIATRIC FDA INDICATIONS:
Seizures.

ADULT FDA INDICATIONS:
Seizure disorders.

OFF-LABEL USES:
Bipolar disorder.

DOSAGE FORMS:
- **Tablets (G):** 150 mg, 300 mg, 600 mg (scored).
- **Oral suspension (G):** 300 mg/5 mL.
- **ER tablets (Oxtellar XR):** 150 mg, 300 mg, 600 mg.

PEDIATRIC DOSAGE GUIDANCE:
- Start 8–10 mg/kg/day divided BID, increase by 5 mg/kg/day in weekly intervals to usual 600–900 mg/day divided BID; max 2400 mg/day.
- No data on use of XR for bipolar disorder; caution as higher doses of XR likely needed when converting from IR to XR (not interchangeable on dose-for-dose basis).

MONITORING: Electrolytes (sodium), HLA-B*1502 in Asians.

COST: IR: $; ER: $$$$$

SIDE EFFECTS:
- Most common: Dizziness, somnolence, headache, ataxia, nausea, vomiting.
- Serious but rare: Potentially serious, sometimes fatal, dermatologic reactions (eg, Stevens-Johnson syndrome, toxic epidermal necrolysis) reported; monitor for skin reactions. Rare cases of anaphylaxis and angioedema reported, even after initial dosing; permanently discontinue should symptoms occur.
- Use caution in patients with previous hypersensitivity to carbamazepine (cross-sensitivity occurs in 25%–30%). Clinically significant hyponatremia (serum sodium <125 mmol/L) may develop (1%–3%; higher rate than with carbamazepine); monitor serum sodium, particularly during the first three months of therapy, especially in patients at risk for hyponatremia.

MECHANISM, PHARMACOKINETICS, AND DRUG INTERACTIONS:
- Sodium channel blocker and neuronal membrane stabilizer.
- Metabolized primarily through CYP450; potent inducer of CYP3A4 and inhibitor of CYP2C19; t ½: 2 hours (9 hours for active metabolite).
- No auto-induction of metabolism and fewer interactions than with carbamazepine. Avoid concomitant use with medications metabolized by CYP3A4 since oxcarbazepine may reduce their levels. Reduces efficacy of oral contraceptives; try nonhormonal measures.

EVIDENCE AND CLINICAL PEARLS:
- In a double-blind study in pediatric mania, it was not statistically better than placebo.
- Oxcarbazepine is the 10-keto analog of carbamazepine (its "chemical cousin"); it is thought of as a gentler carbamazepine due to its more favorable side effect and drug interaction profile.
- Not bioequivalent to carbamazepine. Increase total daily dose by 20%–30% if switching from carbamazepine to oxcarbazepine.
- Screen and avoid using in patients of Asian descent who have HLA-B*1502 allele; risk of Stevens-Johnson syndrome and/or toxic epidermal necrolysis.

FUN FACT:
Synthesized in 1965, oxcarbazepine appeared on the US market in 2000. In 2010, Novartis pled guilty to marketing it for non-FDA-approved uses, eg, neuropathic pain and bipolar disorder.

VALPROIC ACID (Depakote) Fact Sheet [G]

BOTTOM LINE:
Along with lithium, valproate is a first-line antimanic agent for acute manic episodes in kids. Avoid in patients with ovaries due to risk of PCOS as well as risk of congenital malformation; if used, ensure adequate contraception (ideally IUD or depot contraceptive).

PEDIATRIC FDA INDICATIONS:
Seizures.

ADULT FDA INDICATIONS:
Seizures; bipolar disorder (acute mania); migraine prophylaxis.

OFF-LABEL USES:
Bipolar maintenance; impulse control disorders; violence and aggression.

DOSAGE FORMS:
- **Capsules (valproic acid, [G]):** 250 mg.
- **Oral liquid (Depakene, [G]):** 250 mg/5 mL.
- **Delayed-release tablets (Depakote, [G]):** 125 mg, 250 mg, 500 mg.
- **Delayed-release capsules (Depakote Sprinkles, [G]):** 125 mg.
- **ER tablets (Depakote ER, [G]):** 250 mg, 500 mg.

PEDIATRIC DOSAGE GUIDANCE:
- Start 15 mg/kg/day divided BID–TID, increase by 5–10 mg/kg/day in weekly intervals; max 60 mg/kg/day. Typical dosing range in kids is 500–2000 mg/day divided BID–TID.
- When converting from regular Depakote to Depakote ER, be aware that patients will get about 20% less valproic acid with the ER formulation. ER better tolerated when dosed once daily in the morning.

MONITORING: LFTs, CBC for platelets, lipids, pregnancy test, weight, serum drug level, ammonia in patients with confusion, and amylase and lipase when pancreatitis is suspected.

COST: $

SIDE EFFECTS:
- Most common: Somnolence, nausea, fatigue, dizziness, hair loss, tremor, thrombocytopenia (up to 24% of patients; dose-related; reversible).
- Serious but rare: Hepatotoxicity—rare idiosyncratic reaction, not dose-related; most cases occur within three months; risk factors: age <2 years, multiple anticonvulsants, and presence of neurologic disease in addition to epilepsy. Asymptomatic elevations of liver enzymes may occur, not necessarily associated with hepatic dysfunction. Pancreatitis (rare but potentially fatal). Polycystic ovary syndrome (PCOS) in about 10% of genetically born females. Hyperammonemia, encephalopathy (sometimes fatal) reported and may present with normal liver enzymes.

MECHANISM, PHARMACOKINETICS, AND DRUG INTERACTIONS:
- Sodium channel blocker.
- Metabolized primarily by liver with only minimal (10%) role of CYP450 enzymes (2A6, 2B6, 2C9); t ½: 9–16 hours.
- VPA causes ↑ levels of lamotrigine and risk for rash. Taking with topiramate can lead to encephalopathy.

EVIDENCE AND CLINICAL PEARLS:
- Significantly more data in pediatric bipolar than other agents, with eight open-label studies (average response rate: 43%) and three double-blind studies, one of which did not separate from placebo.
- Once steady-state levels reached (within two to four days of initiation or dose adjustment), trough serum levels should be drawn just before the next dose (21–24 hours post-dose for ER/DR preparations) or before the morning dose (12 hours for immediate-release preparations). Target serum level: 50–125 mcg/mL.
- Valproate often reduces available carnitine, which is needed for cell transport physiology. This results in elevated ammonia levels, creating fatigue, confusion, and other symptoms of metabolic stress. Carnitine can be very safely replaced using a minimum twice-daily dosing of carnitine in 330 mg capsules (can be opened, but contents have a strong odor) and titrating up based on repeat laboratory studies.

FUN FACT:
Valproic acid was first synthesized in 1882 by B. S. Burton as an analogue of valeric acid, found naturally in valerian.

Mood Stabilizers

Substance Use Medications

The primary treatment of substance use disorders in teens remains behavioral therapies, particularly motivational interviewing, as well as harm reduction measures. The barriers to care for substance use are higher in adolescents than adults. While substance use medications are likely effective in adolescents, data remain sparse. Only buprenorphine is FDA approved for adolescents age 16 and up, and it is infrequently offered despite its demonstrated efficacy. For other medications, use adult indications and dosing recommendations as a guide. And be sure to address comorbid mental health conditions, specifically ADHD, because treating such kids with stimulants may decrease the risk of substance use.

ALCOHOL USE DISORDERS

While not often used in adolescents, three medications are approved in adults for alcohol use. Acamprosate can be useful in reducing cravings and for maintaining abstinence through its modulating effects on the glutamate system. Disulfiram inhibits the breakdown of alcohol by inhibiting alcohol dehydrogenase, which leads to headaches, flushing, nausea, and tachycardia in those who drink while taking the medication. Disulfiram cannot be started until 12–36 hours after the last drink, and adherence can be low—so, given the impulsivity of adolescents who are drinking, disulfiram is unlikely to be appropriate in most patients. Naltrexone acts on an opioid receptor to blunt the pleasurable effects of alcohol as well as decrease cravings. Topiramate, though not FDA approved for this use, is effective in reducing alcohol craving in adults.

CANNABIS USE DISORDERS

Cannabis options have increased exponentially as more states have legalized marijuana, with more potent options available that can exacerbate negative sequelae. Families may ask about pharmacologic treatment options. N-acetylcysteine (NAC) and topiramate have been studied in adolescents in small randomized, double-blind, placebo-controlled trials. NAC was associated with higher rates of negative urine cannabinoid tests, while topiramate was not associated with improved abstinence but did have lower reports of quantity used. It is important to address comorbidities of depression and anxiety.

NICOTINE USE DISORDERS

Nicotine replacement therapies are available in many forms and may help with weaning adolescents off of nicotine. While concerns about the effects of continued nicotine exposure on a developing brain are valid, the harm reduction benefits of nicotine replacement therapy are clear. Obtain a thorough history to calculate daily nicotine use, using the guideline that one pack per day = 21 mg. The patch should be placed in different positions at the same time each day to avoid skin irritation, used for one to two months, then tapered every one to two months as tolerated. Gum and lozenges can help for fast relief when needed while on the patch. Nicotine patches and gum are available over the counter for adults only, so you'll have to write out a prescription for those under 18. Bupropion is effective for smoking cessation in adults, with limited data that demonstrate efficacy in adolescents. Varenicline can help decrease cravings in adults, but data in adolescents thus far have not consistently demonstrated efficacy, so we don't recommend it as a first-line option.

OPIOID USE DISORDERS

Naltrexone is an opioid antagonist that you can start after your patient completes detox, and it works by preventing the opioid from causing euphoria. Buprenorphine has a few adolescent studies that demonstrate efficacy in decreasing withdrawal and cravings, reducing opioid use, as well as having higher engagement in treatment. Due to the passage of the Mainstreaming Addiction Treatment (MAT) Act on December 29, 2022 in the US, the DEA X-waiver will no longer be required to prescribe buprenorphine, removing a significant barrier for patients. The Medication Access and Training Expansion (MATE) Act, which passed along with the MAT Act, will require that all healthcare providers who apply for or seek renewal of their DEA number take an eight-hour government-approved course in understanding and treating addiction. Monthly office-based maintenance treatment is available, which provides more flexibility than methadone maintenance. Methadone is an opioid agonist that can be used as a substitute for other opiates, but it has limited effect in achieving sobriety. Some states allow older adolescents who have failed other treatments to receive methadone treatment with the consent of their guardian. It comes with the onerous requirement of presenting daily to the methadone clinic in order to receive a dose, which can be very limiting with regard to vocational, academic, and family schedules. Naloxone is now more readily available to families and emergency service personnel to reverse opioid overdose and prevent deaths, and can be obtained without a prescription. Any patient that is prescribed an opiate or has an opioid use disorder should be provided a prescription for naloxone. Finally, fentanyl strips are more available for people to detect the presence of this deadly synthetic opiate, which is routinely cut into heroin and other opiates, including black-market oxycodone pills.

How Long to Treat?

Methadone treatment is typically chronic, and while early recommendations for buprenorphine planned for gradual discontinuation, patients with opioid use disorders typically require long-term medication treatment.

OTHER DRUGS

There are currently no FDA-approved medications in adults or adolescents to address cocaine, benzodiazepine, methamphetamine, or cannabis use, so we haven't included fact sheets for some medications addressing these specific issues. However, you might find the Carlat Psychiatry Guidebook, *Addiction Treatment* by Michael Weaver, MD, a useful resource.

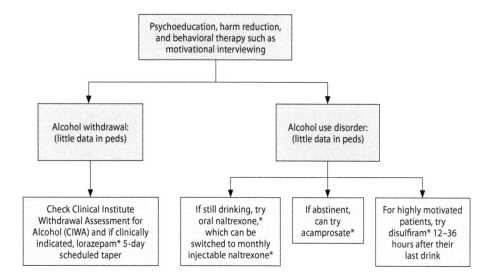

Alcohol Use Disorder Treatment Algorithm for Children and Adolescents

*Denotes off label

Psychoeducation, harm reduction, and behavioral therapy such as motivational interviewing

Alcohol withdrawal: (little data in peds)

Alcohol use disorder: (little data in peds)

Check Clinical Institute Withdrawal Assessment for Alcohol (CIWA) and if clinically indicated, lorazepam* 5-day scheduled taper

If still drinking, try oral naltrexone,* which can be switched to monthly injectable naltrexone*

If abstinent, can try acamprosate*

For highly motivated patients, try disulfiram* 12–36 hours after their last drink

- Use non-pharmacologic approaches first when possible to help reduce use of medication
- See text and tables for specific age-related guidance
- If stable, use clinical judgment to consider gradual taper and discontinuation of medications

CARLAT PUBLISHING © 2023

Nicotine Use Disorder Treatment Algorithm for Children and Adolescents

*Denotes off label

Psychoeducation, harm reduction, and behavioral therapy such as motivational interviewing

Nicotine substitution therapy (limited data in pediatrics): Try nicotine patch (1 PPD = 21 mg patch)*

If cravings continue with patch, add nicotine gum/lozenge* PRN

If comorbid depression/ADHD: Add bupropion*

Varenicline*

- Use non-pharmacologic approaches first when possible to help reduce use of medication
- See text and tables for specific age-related guidance
- If using antidepressants, discuss potential side effects including rare but possible increase in behavioral activation or suicidal thinking
- If stable, use clinical judgment to consider gradual taper and discontinuation of medications

Opioid Use Disorder Treatment Algorithm for Children and Adolescents

*Denotes off label

Psychoeducation, harm reduction, including providing naloxone, and behavioral therapy such as motivational interviewing

Opioid substitution therapy, check Clinical Opiate Withdrawal Scale (COWS)

Buprenorphine/naloxone* | Methadone*

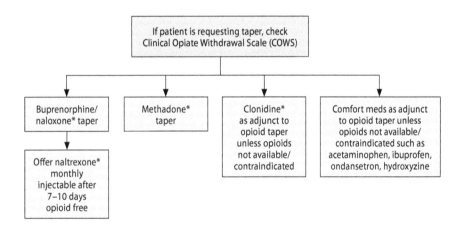

If patient is requesting taper, check Clinical Opiate Withdrawal Scale (COWS)

- Buprenorphine/naloxone* taper
  - Offer naltrexone* monthly injectable after 7–10 days opioid free
- Methadone* taper
- Clonidine* as adjunct to opioid taper unless opioids not available/contraindicated
- Comfort meds as adjunct to opioid taper unless opioids not available/contraindicated such as acetaminophen, ibuprofen, ondansetron, hydroxyzine

- Use non-pharmacologic approaches first when possible to help reduce use of medication
- See text and tables for specific age-related guidance
- General guidance supports ongoing maintenance treatment; use clinical judgment if considering gradual taper or discontinuation of medications

CARLAT PUBLISHING © 2023

TABLE 12: Substance Use Disorder Medications

Generic Name (Brand Name) Year FDA Approved (Rx status) [G] denotes generic availability	Relevant FDA Indication(s)	Available Strengths (mg)	Usual Adult Dosage Range (mg)
Acamprosate [G] (Campral) 2004 (Rx)	Alcohol	333	666 TID
Buprenorphine [G] (Belbuca, Buprenex, Butrans, Subutex) 2002 (C-III)	**Opioid (16+ yrs)**	2, 8 SL (Subutex, [G]) 0.075, 0.15, 0.3, 0.45, 0.6, 0.75, 0.9 buccal film (Belbuca, [G]) (used for pain) 0.3 mg/mL inj (Buprenex, [G]) (used for pain) 5, 7.5, 10, 15, 20 mcg/hr patch (Butrans) (used for pain)	8–16 QD
Buprenorphine extended-release injection (Sublocade) 2017 (C-III)	Opioid	100, 300	300 monthly ×2 doses, then 100 monthly
Buprenorphine/naloxone [G] (Bunavail, Suboxone, Zubsolv) 2002 (C-III) Generic available for 2/0.5, 8/2 mg SL tablets and film strips only	**Opioid (16+ yrs)**	2.1/0.3, 4.2/0.7, 6.3/1 buccal film (Bunavail) 2/0.5, 4/1, 8/2, 12/3 SL film strips (Suboxone, [G]) 2/0.5, 8/2 SL tabs (generic only) 0.7/0.18, 1.4/0.36, 2.9/0.71, 5.7/1.4, 8.6/2.1, 11.4/2.9 SL tabs (Zubsolv)	4–24 QD
Bupropion SR [G] (Zyban) 1997 (Rx)	Smoking	150	150 QAM–150 BID
Disulfiram [G] (Antabuse) 1951 (Rx)	Alcohol	250, 500	125–500 QPM
Methadone [G] (Dolophine, Methadose) 1947 (C-II)	Opioid	5, 10, 40 10 mg/mL, 10 mg/5 mL, 5 mg/5 mL oral liquid	20–120 QD
Naloxone [G] (Narcan Nasal Spray, Kloxxado, Zimhi) 2015 (intranasal) (Rx)	Emergency opioid overdose rescue	4 mg/0.1 mL (Narcan), 8 mg/0.1 mL (Kloxxado) intranasal 5 mg/0.5 mL intramuscular or subcutaneous (Zimhi)	*IV/IM/SC:* Infants and children ≤5 years or ≤20 kg: 0.1 mg/kg/dose. Children >5 years or >20 kg and adolescents: 2 mg/dose. *Intranasal:* 4 mg or 8 mg ×1, repeat every 2–3 minutes.
Naltrexone [G] (ReVia) 1984 (Rx)	Alcohol, opioid	50	25–50 QD
Naltrexone ER (Vivitrol) 2006 (Rx)	Alcohol, opioid	380	380 Q4 weeks
Nicotine inhaled (Nicotrol Inhaler) 1997 (Rx)	Smoking	4 mg delivered/cartridge	6–16 cartridges/day

Generic Name (Brand Name) Year FDA Approved (Rx status) [G] denotes generic availability	Relevant FDA Indication(s)	Available Strengths (mg)	Usual Adult Dosage Range (mg)
Nicotine nasal spray (Nicotrol NS) 1996 (Rx)	Smoking	0.5 mg delivered/spray	1–2 sprays/hour PRN
Nicotine polacrilex [G] (Nicorette Gum, others) 1992 (OTC; Rx if <18 yrs)	Smoking	2, 4	1 piece PRN up to 24/day
Nicotine polacrilex [G] (Nicorette Lozenge, others) 2009 (OTC; Rx if <18 yrs)	Smoking	2, 4	1 piece PRN up to 20/day
Nicotine transdermal [G] (Habitrol, Nicoderm CQ) 1991 (OTC; Rx if <18 yrs)	Smoking	7, 14, 21/24 hours	14–21 QD
Varenicline (Chantix) 2006 (Rx)	Smoking	0.5, 1	0.5 QD–1 BID

ACAMPROSATE (Campral) Fact Sheet [G]

BOTTOM LINE:
Acamprosate and naltrexone show similar reduced rates of relapse, but acamprosate is associated with more diarrhea, while naltrexone is associated with more nausea, fatigue, and somnolence; acamprosate is preferred in patients with hepatic impairment. Limited data in children but seems to be well tolerated.

PEDIATRIC FDA INDICATIONS:
None.

ADULT FDA INDICATIONS:
Alcohol dependence.

OFF-LABEL USES:
None.

DOSAGE FORMS:
Delayed-release tablets (G): 333 mg.

DOSAGE GUIDANCE (ADULTS):
Start 666 mg TID. Give 333 mg TID in patients with renal impairment.

MONITORING: BUN/creatinine.

COST: $$

SIDE EFFECTS:
- Most common: Diarrhea (dose-related, transient), flatulence, weakness, peripheral edema, insomnia, anxiety.
- Serious but rare: Acute renal failure reported in a few cases; suicidal ideation, attempts, and completions rare but greater than with placebo in studies.

MECHANISM, PHARMACOKINETICS, AND DRUG INTERACTIONS:
- Mechanism of action is not fully defined; it appears to work by promoting a balance between the excitatory and inhibitory neurotransmitters, glutamate and GABA, respectively (GABA and glutamate activities appear to be disrupted in alcohol dependence).
- Not metabolized, cleared as unchanged drug by kidneys; t ½: 20–33 hours.
- There are no significant drug interactions.

EVIDENCE AND CLINICAL PEARLS:
- Clinically, acamprosate has demonstrated efficacy in more than 25 placebo-controlled trials in adults, and it has generally been found to be more effective than placebo in reducing risk of returning to any drinking and increasing the cumulative duration of abstinence. However, in reducing heavy drinking, acamprosate appears to be no better than placebo.
- Clinical data in adolescents with alcohol use disorder are limited but promising. Additional studies in autistic children and fragile X syndrome have found acamprosate to be generally safe and well tolerated in the pediatric population.
- Acamprosate can be used with naltrexone or disulfiram (different mechanism of action), although the combination with naltrexone may not increase efficacy per available studies.
- Approved by the FDA in 2004, but it has been used in France and other countries since 1989.
- Does not eliminate or treat symptoms of alcohol withdrawal. Usually prescribed for maintenance of abstinence; may continue even if patient relapses with alcohol.
- Taking with food is not necessary, but it may help compliance to do so.
- Compared to naltrexone and disulfiram, acamprosate is unique in that it is not metabolized by the liver and is not impacted by alcohol use, so it can be administered to patients with hepatitis or liver disease and to patients who continue drinking alcohol.

FUN FACT:
Each 333 mg tablet contains 33 mg of elemental calcium (because it is available as acamprosate calcium salt).

BUPRENORPHINE (Sublocade) Fact Sheet [G]

BOTTOM LINE:
Buprenorphine alone was previously preferred for initial (induction) phase of treatment, with buprenorphine/naloxone combination preferred for maintenance treatment (unsupervised administration). Currently, combination is favored for both induction and maintenance as this decreases misuse or diversion potential. Studied and approved for ages ≥16.

PEDIATRIC FDA INDICATIONS:
Pain (2+ years).

ADULT FDA INDICATIONS (16+ YEARS):
Opioid dependence, induction; opioid dependence, maintenance (Sublocade); moderate-severe pain (Belbuca, Buprenex, Butrans).

OFF-LABEL USES:
None.

DOSAGE FORMS:
- **SL tablets (G):** 2 mg, 8 mg (scored).
- **Extended-release injection (Sublocade):** 100 mg/0.5 mL, 300 mg/1.5 mL prefilled syringes.
- **Buccal film (Belbuca, [G]):** 0.075 mg, 0.15 mg, 0.3 mg, 0.45 mg, 0.6 mg, 0.75 mg, 0.9 mg (used for pain).
- **Injection (Buprenex, [G]):** 0.3 mg/mL (used for pain).
- **Transdermal patch (Butrans):** 5 mcg/hr, 7.5 mcg/hr, 10 mcg/hr, 15 mcg/hr, 20 mcg/hr (used for pain).

DOSAGE GUIDANCE (16+ YEARS):
- Begin at least four hours after last use of heroin or other short-acting opioids and when first signs of withdrawal appear. If an opioid-dependent patient is not in sufficient withdrawal, introduction of buprenorphine may precipitate withdrawal due to its partial agonist effect.
- Start 2–8 mg SL day 1; then 8–16 mg SL QD (usual induction dose range is 12–16 mg/day and accomplished over three to four days).
- Other than extended-release injection, not for maintenance treatment; patients should be switched to the buprenorphine/naloxone combination for maintenance and unsupervised therapy.
- Patients with moderate to severe opioid use disorder and stabilized with SL or buccal buprenorphine for >7 days may convert to monthly subcutaneous injections. Start 300 mg monthly for two months, then 100 mg monthly maintenance. Some patients may require higher doses.

MONITORING: LFTs.

COST: SL: $$; monthly injection: $$$$$

SIDE EFFECTS:
- Most common: Headache, pain, insomnia, nausea, anxiety.
- Serious but rare: Hepatitis reported rarely, ranging from transient, asymptomatic transaminase elevations to hepatic failure; in many cases, patients had preexisting hepatic dysfunction. QT prolongation with higher doses of transdermal.

MECHANISM, PHARMACOKINETICS, AND DRUG INTERACTIONS:
- Opioid agonist (delta and mu receptors) and antagonist (kappa receptors).
- Metabolized primarily through CYP3A4; t ½: 24–48 hours.
- Avoid concomitant use with opiate analgesics: diminished pain control. Additive effects with CNS depressants. CYP3A4 inhibitors and inducers may affect levels of buprenorphine.

EVIDENCE AND CLINICAL PEARLS:
- C-III controlled substance. Prescribing of SL tablets for opioid dependence will no longer be limited to prescribers with a DEA X-waiver. Moving forward, all prescribers renewing or applying for their DEA number will be required to take an eight-hour substance use treatment course and will be able to prescribe buprenorphine.
- Previously, there were limits to the number of patients an X-waivered provider could treat with buprenophine. As of this book's publishing date, such limits are no longer expected.
- Binds to various opioid receptors, producing agonism at delta receptors, partial agonism at mu receptors, and antagonism at kappa receptors (opioid agonist-antagonist).
- Although only studied in adults thus far, monthly injection offers alternative that may be convenient for some patients.

FUN FACT:
The subcutaneous implant formulation of buprenorphine (Probuphine) was discontinued. Its use was severely limited as it was invasive, expensive, and an option only for patients stable on ≤8 mg/day. Other implants currently in development include medications that will treat schizophrenia, breast cancer, photosensitivity, and Parkinson's disease.

BUPRENORPHINE/NALOXONE (Bunavail, Suboxone, Zubsolv) Fact Sheet [G]

BOTTOM LINE:
The combination product is preferred over buprenorphine alone for maintenance because the addition of naloxone affords it a lower potential for injection misuse. The SL film formulation is priced a little higher than the SL tablets, yet provides very little (if any) meaningful benefits; generic SL tablets should be used as a cost-saving measure.

PEDIATRIC FDA INDICATIONS:
None.

ADULT FDA INDICATIONS (16+ YEARS):
Opioid dependence (induction and maintenance); approved for adolescents aged 16+.

OFF-LABEL USES:
None.

DOSAGE FORMS:
- **SL tablets (G):** 2/0.5 mg, 8/2 mg (scored).
- **SL film strips (Suboxone, [G]):** 2/0.5 mg, 4/1 mg, 8/2 mg, 12/3 mg.
- **SL tablets (Zubsolv):** 0.7/0.18 mg, 1.4/0.36 mg, 2.9/0.71 mg, 5.7/1.4 mg, 8.6/2.1 mg, 11.4/2.9 mg.
- **Buccal film (Bunavail):** 2.1/0.3 mg, 4.2/0.7 mg, 6.3/1 mg.

DOSAGE GUIDANCE (16+ YEARS):
- For induction, use strategy described in buprenorphine fact sheet. For maintenance, give combination product (Suboxone or [G]) daily in the equivalent buprenorphine dose on last day of induction; adjust dose in increments of 2 mg or 4 mg to a level that maintains treatment and suppresses opioid withdrawal symptoms (usually 4–24 mg/day); max 32 mg/day.
- Zubsolv 5.7/1.4 mg SL tablet provides equivalent buprenorphine to a Suboxone 8/2 mg SL tablet.
- Bunavail 4.2/0.7 mg buccal film provides equivalent buprenorphine to a Suboxone 8/2 mg SL tablet.

MONITORING: LFTs.

COST: SL tablet, film, Bunavail: $–$$ depending on dose; Zubsolv: $$$$$

SIDE EFFECTS:
- Most common: Headache, pain, vomiting, sweating.
- Serious but rare: Hepatitis reported rarely, ranging from transient, asymptomatic transaminase elevations to hepatic failure; in many cases, patients had preexisting hepatic dysfunction.

MECHANISM, PHARMACOKINETICS, AND DRUG INTERACTIONS:
- Buprenorphine: opioid agonist (delta and mu receptors) and antagonist (kappa receptors); naloxone: opioid antagonist.
- Metabolized primarily through CYP3A4; t ½: 24–48 hours (naloxone: 2–12 hours).
- Avoid concomitant use with opiate analgesics: diminished pain control. Additive effects with CNS depressants. CYP3A4 inhibitors and inducers may affect levels of buprenorphine.

EVIDENCE AND CLINICAL PEARLS:
- Two randomized controlled trials in adolescents and young adults, with some kids as young as 13, found buprenorphine to be safe and effective.
- C-III controlled substance. Prescribing of SL tablets for opioid dependence will no longer be limited to prescribers with a DEA X-waiver. Moving forward, all prescribers renewing or applying for their DEA number will be required to take an eight-hour substance use treatment course and will be able to prescribe buprenorphine.
- Previously, there were limits to the number of patients an X-waivered provider could treat with buprenophine. As of this book's publishing date, such limits are no longer expected.
- Naloxone is an opioid antagonist that is active only when injected; it is added to buprenorphine in order to reduce misuse via intravenous injection of a dissolved tablet.
- The SL film formulation's manufacturer claims it dissolves faster and tastes better than SL tablets. Actually, it is more likely a way for the manufacturer to switch users to a "new" product (with patent protection until 2025) rather than lose patients to generics.
- SL film should be placed at base of tongue to the side of midline; this allows patient to use two films at the same time if dose dictates.
- Zubsolv and Bunavail formulations have better bioavailability, hence the dose equivalencies noted above.
- Prescribers should be aware of the high risk for diversion and sale of buprenorphine films and tablets. Some regular opioid users periodically buy buprenorphine "off the street" and use it to combat cravings and withdrawal symptoms if their drug of choice is not readily available.

FUN FACT:
The manufacturer of Suboxone, Reckitt Benckiser, generates most of its revenue from selling home and personal care products like Lysol cleaners and Durex condoms.

DISULFIRAM (Antabuse) Fact Sheet [G]

BOTTOM LINE:
Disulfiram is an aversive treatment, causing a buildup of ethanol's metabolite acetaldehyde in the serum, which in turn causes symptoms such as flushing, dizziness, nausea, and vomiting. Since craving is not reduced by disulfiram and any alcohol ingestion could result in a reaction, nonadherence can be common. Its use should be reserved for selective, highly motivated, and thoroughly informed patients in conjunction with supportive and psychotherapeutic treatment.

PEDIATRIC FDA INDICATIONS:
None.

ADULT FDA INDICATIONS:
Alcohol dependence.

OFF-LABEL USES:
None.

DOSAGE FORMS:
Tablets (G): 250 mg, 500 mg.

DOSAGE GUIDANCE (ADULTS):
Start 125 mg QPM (must be abstinent from alcohol >12 hours), increase to 250 mg QPM after several days. Maintenance is usually 250–500 mg QPM, but some patients can drink alcohol without a reaction at the 250 mg/day dose.

MONITORING: LFTs.

COST: $

SIDE EFFECTS:
- Most common: Skin eruptions (eg, acne, allergic dermatitis), drowsiness, fatigue, impotence, headache, metallic taste.
- Serious but rare: Severe (very rarely fatal) hepatitis or hepatic failure has been reported and may occur in patients with or without prior history of abnormal hepatic function. Rare psychotic episodes have been reported. Rarely may cause peripheral neuropathy or optic neuritis.

MECHANISM, PHARMACOKINETICS, AND DRUG INTERACTIONS:
- Aldehyde dehydrogenase inhibitor.
- Metabolized primarily through CYP450; t ½: not defined, but elimination from body is slow, and effects may persist for one or two weeks after last dose.
- While taking disulfiram, and for one to two weeks after stopping, avoid concomitant use of any medications containing alcohol (including topicals), metronidazole, or "disguised" forms of ethanol (cough syrup, some mouthwashes, oral solutions or liquid concentrates containing alcohol such as sertraline). Avoid vinegars, cider, extracts, and foods containing ethanol.

EVIDENCE AND CLINICAL PEARLS:
- Disulfiram has been studied and benefit has been shown in adolescents. Use in adolescents may be even riskier than in adults given adolescents' impulsivity and risk-taking behaviors, somewhat limiting disulfiram's appropriateness in this population.
- Disulfiram inhibits the enzyme aldehyde dehydrogenase; when taken with alcohol, acetaldehyde levels are increased by five- to 10-fold, causing unpleasant symptoms that include flushing, nausea, vomiting, palpitations, chest pain, vertigo, hypotension, and (in rare instances) cardiovascular collapse and death. This is the basis for its use as aversion therapy. Common advice to patients: "You'll wish you were dead, but it likely won't kill you."
- Reaction may last from 30–60 minutes to several hours or as long as alcohol remains in the bloodstream.
- Advise patients to carry an identification card or a medical alert bracelet that states they are taking the medication and lists the symptoms of the reaction and clinician contact information.
- Duration of therapy is until the patient is fully recovered and a basis for permanent self-control has been established; maintenance therapy may be required for months or even years.

FUN FACT:
Disulfiram's antiprotozoal activity may be effective in *Giardia* and *Trichomonas* infections.

METHADONE (Methadose) Fact Sheet [G]

BOTTOM LINE:
Opioid replacement therapy via methadone reduces or eliminates illicit use of opioids and criminality associated with opioid use, supporting health and social functioning. It is a harm reduction model reducing transmission of infectious diseases such as hepatitis and HIV. Disadvantages include potential for accumulation with repeated doses (which may result in toxicity), interindividual variability in pharmacokinetic parameters, potential for drug interactions, challenges associated with dose titration, stigma associated with opioid replacement therapy, and limited availability of treatment programs (nonexistent in some geographic areas, long wait lists in other areas). Methadone has long been established as an effective treatment of opioid addiction in adults, although federal regulations prohibit most methadone programs from admitting patients younger than 18 years.

PEDIATRIC FDA INDICATIONS:
None.

ADULT FDA INDICATIONS:
Opioid dependence; severe pain.

OFF-LABEL USES:
None.

DOSAGE FORMS:
- **Tablets (G):** 5 mg, 10 mg, 40 mg (scored),
- **Oral solution (G):** 5 mg/5 mL, 10 mg/5 mL.
- **Oral concentrate (G):** 10 mg/mL.

DOSAGE GUIDANCE (ADULTS):
Start 15–30 mg single dose; then 5–10 mg every two to four hours. Adjust dose to prevent withdrawal symptoms; max 40 mg on day 1. 80–120 mg per day is a common maintenance dose for opioid dependence.

MONITORING: ECG.

COST: $

SIDE EFFECTS:
- Most common: Constipation, dizziness, sedation, nausea, sweating.
- Serious but rare: May prolong the QT interval and increase risk for torsades de pointes; caution in patients at risk for QT prolongation; usually with doses >100 mg/day. Severe respiratory depression may occur; use extreme caution during initiation, titration, and conversion from other opioids to methadone. Respiratory depressant effects occur later and persist longer than analgesic effects, possibly contributing to cases of overdose.

MECHANISM, PHARMACOKINETICS, AND DRUG INTERACTIONS:
- Opioid agonist.
- Metabolized primarily through CYP2B6, 2C19, and 3A4 (major); inhibits CYP2D6; t ½: 8–59 hours.
- High potential for interactions. Avoid concomitant use with other potent sedatives or respiratory depressants. Use with caution in patients on medications metabolized that are by CYP2D6, inhibit CYP3A4, prolong the QT interval, or promote electrolyte depletion.

EVIDENCE AND CLINICAL PEARLS:
- A few studies in adolescents. Most recently, a 12-month study of 120 adolescents found methadone treatment reduced heroin use, but treatment retention was challenging (similar to adult studies).
- C-II controlled substance; distribution of 40 mg tablets restricted to authorized opioid addiction treatment facilities.
- May only be dispensed according to the Substance Abuse and Mental Health Services Administration's (SAMHSA) Center for Substance Abuse Treatment (CSAT) guidelines. Regulations vary by area; consult regulatory agencies and/or methadone treatment facilities.
- Methadone accumulates with repeated doses; dose may need reduction after three to five days to prevent CNS depressant effects.

FUN FACT:
A persistent but untrue urban legend claims the name "Dolophine" was coined in tribute to Adolf Hitler by its German creators. The name was in fact created after the war by the American branch of Eli Lilly, and the pejorative term "adolphine" (never an actual name of the drug) didn't appear in the US until the early 1970s.

NALOXONE (Kloxxado, Narcan Nasal Spray, Zimhi) Fact Sheet [G]

BOTTOM LINE:
Naloxone rescue saves lives. Prescribe it to all patients and families who have opioids available in their living environments.

PEDIATRIC FDA INDICATIONS:
Emergency treatment of known or suspected opioid overdose.

ADULT FDA INDICATIONS:
Emergency treatment of known or suspected opioid overdose.

OFF-LABEL USES:
None.

DOSAGE FORMS:
- **Intranasal (Narcan Nasal Spray):** 4 mg/0.1 mL.
- **Intranasal (Kloxxado):** 8 mg/0.1 mL.
- **Injectable prefilled syringe (Zimhi):** 5 mg/0.5 mL.
- Generic intranasal kit may be assembled using 2 mg/2 mL prefilled needleless syringe and a mucosal atomization device nasal adapter (requires assembly at time of administration).

PEDIATRIC DOSAGE GUIDANCE:
- IV/IM/SC: Infants and children ≤5 years or ≤20 kg: 0.1 mg/kg/dose; repeat every two to three minutes if needed; may need to repeat doses every 20–60 minutes.
- IV/IM/SC: Children >5 years or >20 kg and adolescents: 2 mg/dose; if no response, repeat every two to three minutes; may need to repeat doses every 20–60 minutes.
- Intranasal: 4 mg or 8 mg x1 spray in one nostril. Bystander to spray in one nostril; may repeat into other nostril with additional doses every two to three minutes if no or minimal response and until emergency response arrives. The drug is absorbed automatically into the nasal mucosa.

MONITORING: No specific monitoring of note.

COST: 4 mg intranasal, generic kit: $; 8 mg intranasal, Zimhi: $$$

SIDE EFFECTS:
Most common: Symptoms of opioid withdrawal, including body aches, fever, sweating, runny nose, sneezing, piloerection, yawning, weakness, shivering or trembling, nervousness, restlessness or irritability, diarrhea, nausea or vomiting, abdominal cramps, increased blood pressure, and tachycardia.

MECHANISM, PHARMACOKINETICS, AND DRUG INTERACTIONS:
- Opioid antagonist.
- Metabolized primarily by conjugation (non-P450) in the liver; t ½: 1.36 hours.

EVIDENCE AND CLINICAL PEARLS:
- No studies specifically in kids or adolescents, but clinical use in opioid overdose situations is the same as in adults.
- Because treatment of overdose with this opioid antagonist must be performed by someone other than the patient, instruct the prescription recipient to inform local acquaintances about having naloxone rescue and ensure that they have been instructed in recognition of overdose symptoms and naloxone administration.
- Zimhi is a new injectable (intramuscular or subcutaneous) prefilled syringe for layperson use but comes in a much higher 5 mg dose and delivers nearly five-fold higher peak serum concentrations, which could result in very severe precipitated withdrawal symptoms.
- Like Zimhi, Kloxxado is a higher-dose formulation that was developed to combat the presumed need for repeated doses of naloxone after overdose with higher-potency opioids such as fentanyl. Whether multiple doses are required has been controversial, and use of this ultra-potent antagonist could result in severe precipitated withdrawal. Kloxxado is likely overkill for most patients—stick to the 4 mg nasal formulation.
- Most opioids have a longer duration of action than naloxone, so overdose symptoms (CNS and respiratory depression) may return after initial improvement. Patients should receive medical attention and continue to be monitored after provision of emergency dose(s).
- Check out the Prescribe to Prevent website (www.prescribetoprevent.org) for prescriber resources such as webinars, toolkits, patient education materials, and medical-legal resources. This website also provides guidance to physicians on writing a prescription for naloxone.

FUN FACT:
Naloxone was first approved for opioid overdose treatment in 1971 and is available as a very inexpensive injectable generic. These newer formulations will come at a much higher price because of the way they are formulated, making them easier to use by bystanders who are not emergency providers.

NALTREXONE (ReVia, Vivitrol) Fact Sheet [G]

BOTTOM LINE:
Naltrexone, an opioid antagonist, is the first-line medication for alcohol use disorder—though it is also approved for opioid use disorder. By reducing the endorphin-mediated euphoria of drinking, it helps people moderate, preventing that first drink from leading to several more. Avoid it in patients with hepatic impairment or those taking opioids. For opioid dependence, methadone and buprenorphine are more effective for most, although naltrexone may be appropriate for highly motivated opioid-dependent patients, with injectable preferred over oral. Finally, naltrexone is frequently used off label for irritability in autistic kids, often in low 3–5 mg compounded doses.

PEDIATRIC FDA INDICATIONS:
None.

ADULT FDA INDICATIONS:
Alcohol dependence; opioid addiction (relapse prevention following detox).

OFF-LABEL USES:
Self-injurious behavior, irritability in autism.

DOSAGE FORMS:
- **Tablets (ReVia, [G]):** 50 mg (scored).
- **Long-acting injection (Vivitrol):** 380 mg.

DOSAGE GUIDANCE (ADULTS):
- Opioid dependence: Start 25 mg for one day; if no withdrawal signs, increase to and maintain 50 mg/day (with food); doses >50 mg may increase risk of hepatoxicity.
- Alcohol dependence: Start and maintain 50 mg QD.
- Injection: 380 mg IM (gluteal) Q4 weeks (for opioid or alcohol dependence). Do not initiate therapy until patient is opioid-free for at least seven to 10 days (by urinalysis).

MONITORING: LFTs.

COST: Tablet: $; injection: $$$$$

SIDE EFFECTS:
- Most common: Headache, nausea, somnolence, vomiting.
- Serious but rare: Black box warning regarding dose-related hepatocellular injury, with a narrow therapeutic window, about ≤5-fold safe vs hepatotoxic. Discontinue if signs/symptoms of acute hepatitis develop.

MECHANISM, PHARMACOKINETICS, AND DRUG INTERACTIONS:
- Opioid antagonist. No significant interactions other than avoiding use with opioids (see below).
- Metabolized primarily through non-CYP450 pathway; t ½: 4 hours (5–10 days for IM).

EVIDENCE AND CLINICAL PEARLS:
- Efficacy (oral) in adults with alcohol dependence (craving and relapse) is more convincing than in opioid dependence, where craving is not decreased but euphoric effects are blocked. Monthly IM may be more effective than oral at maintaining abstinence in opioid dependence (better medication adherence).
- Naltrexone in adolescents has two very small studies in which it was found to reduce craving and alcohol use.
- May precipitate acute withdrawal (pain, hypertension, sweating, agitation, and irritability) in opioid-using patients; ensure patient is opioid-free for at least seven to 10 days prior to initiating.
- In naltrexone-treated patients requiring emergency pain management, consider alternatives to opioids (eg, regional analgesia, non-opioid analgesics, general anesthesia). If opioid therapy is required, patients should be under the direct care of a trained anesthesia provider.
- In addition to the 25–50 mg doses, smaller compounded amounts of 3–5 mg, called low-dose naltrexone (LDN), are often used for irritability in autistic kids.

FUN FACT:
Methylnaltrexone, a closely related drug, is marketed as Relistor for the treatment of opioid-induced constipation.

NICOTINE GUM/LOZENGE (Nicorette) Fact Sheet [G]

BOTTOM LINE:
First-line intervention for those patients who can stop smoking at initiation of therapy; nicotine in the form of gum or lozenge may act as a substitute oral activity, which may aid in behavior modification. Also a good complement to the nicotine patch for breakthrough withdrawal symptoms or craving.

PEDIATRIC FDA INDICATIONS:
None.

ADULT FDA INDICATIONS:
Smoking cessation.

OFF-LABEL USES:
None.

DOSAGE FORMS:
- **Gum (G):** 2 mg, 4 mg (over the counter).
- **Lozenges (G):** 2 mg, 4 mg (over the counter).

DOSAGE GUIDANCE (ADULTS):
- For gum: Chew one piece of gum PRN urge to smoke, up to 24 pieces/day. Patients who smoke <25 cigarettes/day should start with 2 mg strength; patients smoking ≥25 cigarettes/day should start with 4 mg strength.
- For lozenges: Patients who smoke their first cigarette within 30 minutes of waking should use 4 mg strength; otherwise 2 mg strength is recommended. Do not use more than one lozenge at a time; maximum is five lozenges every six hours or 20 lozenges/day.
- For both gum and lozenges, use the following 12-week dosing schedule:
  – Weeks 1–6: One piece every one to two hours; use at least nine pieces/day to increase chances of quitting
  – Weeks 7–9: One piece every two to four hours
  – Weeks 10–12: One piece every four to eight hours
- Patients should be advised to completely stop smoking upon initiation of therapy.

MONITORING: No specific monitoring of note.

COST: $

SIDE EFFECTS:
Most common: Headache; indigestion; nausea; hiccups; tongue, mouth, and throat irritation or tingling; jaw ache (gum).

MECHANISM, PHARMACOKINETICS, AND DRUG INTERACTIONS:
- Nicotinic-cholinergic receptor agonist.
- Metabolized primarily through liver as well as kidneys and lungs; t ½: 1–2 hours.
- Minimal risk for drug interactions. Successful cessation of smoking may increase serum levels of medications metabolized by CYP1A2 (eg, clozapine, olanzapine, theophylline), which is induced by hydrocarbons in smoke; nicotine itself has no effect.

EVIDENCE AND CLINICAL PEARLS:
- One study in adolescents showed somewhat higher compliance with patch therapy than with gum, but this may vary with patient preference.
- If there are cravings throughout the day even with a patch, add a short-acting agent (gum, lozenge, spray, inhaler). Discuss chewing technique for gum: Chew a few times (about 15 times) to activate the release (the sign is tingling/bad peppery taste), then park between cheek and gum until tingle is gone (about one minute), and switch sides every few minutes. Repeat until most of the tingle is gone (~30 minutes). Each piece is 2 mg or 4 mg and lasts about 30 minutes.
- Lozenges should not be chewed or swallowed; allow to dissolve slowly (~20–30 minutes).
- Each 4 mg lozenge or gum results in 2 mg of absorbed nicotine, equivalent to two cigarettes.

FUN FACT:
Nicotine gum is available in a variety of flavors: fruit, mint, cinnamon, orange, cherry, and "original."

NICOTINE INHALED (Nicotrol Inhaler) Fact Sheet

BOTTOM LINE:
Very high expense and unpleasant side effects make this form of nicotine replacement therapy difficult to recommend as a first-line option since no single therapy has been shown to be more effective than another. While this delivers nicotine in an inhaled fashion like e-cigarettes, it's a safer and regulated delivery device that is devoid of the dangerous chemicals and unknowns of using the unregulated vaping devices.

PEDIATRIC FDA INDICATIONS:
None.

ADULT FDA INDICATIONS:
Smoking cessation.

OFF-LABEL USES:
None.

DOSAGE FORMS:
Cartridges: 4 mg delivered per 10 mg cartridge (prescription required).

DOSAGE GUIDANCE (ADULTS):
- Use frequent continuous puffing for 20 minutes with each cartridge; 80 deep inhalations over 20 minutes releases 4 mg nicotine, of which 2 mg is absorbed. Use 6–16 cartridges per day. Taper after 6–12 weeks of use by gradual dose reduction over 6–12 additional weeks.
- Patients should be advised to completely stop smoking upon initiation of therapy.

MONITORING: No specific monitoring of note.

COST: $$$$

SIDE EFFECTS:
Most common: Headache, mouth/throat irritation, dyspepsia, cough, unpleasant taste, rhinitis, tearing, sneezing.

MECHANISM, PHARMACOKINETICS, AND DRUG INTERACTIONS:
- Nicotinic-cholinergic receptor agonist.
- Metabolized primarily through liver as well as kidneys and lungs; t ½: 1–2 hours.
- Minimal drug interactions. Successful cessation of smoking may increase serum levels of medications metabolized by CYP1A2 (eg, clozapine, olanzapine, theophylline), which is induced by hydrocarbons in smoke; nicotine itself has no effect.

EVIDENCE AND CLINICAL PEARLS:
- No data specifically in kids or adolescents.
- Insert cartridge into inhaler and push hard until it pops into place. Replace mouthpiece and twist the top and bottom so that markings do not line up. Inhale deeply into the back of the throat or puff in short breaths. Nicotine in cartridge is used up after about 20 minutes of active puffing.
- Do not eat or drink 15 minutes before or during use. Puffing lightly rather than inhaling reduces coughing.
- Irritation in the mouth and throat may occur in about 40% of patients; coughing (32%) and rhinitis (23%) are also common. These effects are generally mild and abate with continued use. Use with caution in patients with bronchospastic disease due to potential airway irritation (consider other forms of nicotine replacement).
- Higher ambient temperatures deliver more nicotine; lower temperatures deliver less.
- One cartridge delivers 80 puffs or about 2 mg of absorbed nicotine. Roughly 10 cartridges per day is equivalent to the nicotine of smoking one pack per day.

FUN FACT:
A nicotine inhaler is not really a true inhaler; puffing deposits the nicotine into the mouth, and it is then absorbed in the same manner as the nicotine gum or lozenge preparations.

NICOTINE NASAL SPRAY (Nicotrol NS) Fact Sheet

BOTTOM LINE:
The idea of nasal administration of nicotine is appealing in that it more closely approximates the time course of plasma nicotine levels observed after cigarette smoking than other dosage forms; however, the high cost coupled with unpleasant side effects make this difficult to recommend as a first-line treatment, especially since no one form of nicotine replacement therapy has been shown to be more effective than another.

PEDIATRIC FDA INDICATIONS:
None.

ADULT FDA INDICATIONS:
Smoking cessation.

OFF-LABEL USES:
None.

DOSAGE FORMS:
10 mL bottle: 10 mg/mL delivering 0.5 mg/spray in 200 sprays (prescription required).

DOSAGE GUIDANCE (ADULTS):
* Use one or two sprays/hour as needed; do not exceed more than five doses (10 sprays) per hour. Max dose is 40 doses/day (80 sprays). Each dose (two sprays) contains 1 mg of nicotine.
* After initial eight weeks of treatment, taper dose gradually over four to six weeks.
* Patients should be advised to completely stop smoking upon initiation of therapy.

MONITORING: No specific monitoring of note.

COST: $$$$

SIDE EFFECTS:
Most common: Headache, dyspepsia, rhinitis, nasal irritation, sneezing, coughing.

MECHANISM, PHARMACOKINETICS, AND DRUG INTERACTIONS:
* Nicotinic-cholinergic receptor agonist.
* Metabolized primarily through liver as well as kidneys and lungs; t ½: 1–2 hours.
* Minimal risk for drug interactions. Successful cessation of smoking may increase serum levels of medications metabolized by CYP1A2 (eg, clozapine, olanzapine, theophylline), which is induced by hydrocarbons in smoke; nicotine itself has no effect.

EVIDENCE AND CLINICAL PEARLS:
* Nicotine nasal spray was not well tolerated in a randomized open-label trial with 40 adolescent smokers. More than half (57%) dropped out of the study after only a week. The most common complaints were nasal irritation and burning, and complaints about the taste and smell.
* Prime pump prior to first use. Blow nose gently prior to use. Tilt head back slightly, breathe through mouth, and spray once in each nostril. Do not sniff, swallow, or inhale through nose.
* Moderate to severe nasal irritation in 94% of patients in the first two days of use; severity decreases over time. Nasal congestion and transient changes in sense of smell and taste also reported. Avoid in patients with chronic nasal disorders (eg, allergy, rhinitis, nasal polyps, and sinusitis). Exacerbations of bronchospasm reported in patients with asthma.
* Heavy smokers may well use the maximum amount of 80 sprays/day, meaning they would need a new bottle every two to three days. This can be tremendously and prohibitively expensive.
* Potential for abuse and dependence appears to be greater than with other nicotine replacement therapy.

FUN FACT:
In a published case report (*Am J Psychiatry* 2001), a 54-year-old man who could no longer afford his Nicotrol NS prescription found a commercial source for nicotine on the internet (sold as an insecticide). He purchased 25 g in a 1 g/mL solution for $30, diluted the nicotine solution with distilled water to 10 mg/mL, and then placed the solution into empty spray bottles.

NICOTINE PATCH (Nicoderm CQ) Fact Sheet [G]

BOTTOM LINE:
Nicotine patches are a first-line intervention in patients who are able to quit smoking at initiation of treatment and who are regular and constant smokers.

PEDIATRIC FDA INDICATIONS:
None.

ADULT FDA INDICATIONS:
Smoking cessation.

OFF-LABEL USES:
None.

DOSAGE FORMS:
Transdermal patch (G): 7 mg, 14 mg, 21 mg/24 hours (over the counter).

DOSAGE GUIDANCE (ADULTS):
- Apply new patch every 24 hours (same time each day, usually after awakening) to non-hairy, clean, dry skin on the upper body or upper outer arm; each patch should be applied to a different site. Adjustment may be required during initial treatment (increase dose if experiencing withdrawal symptoms; lower dose if experiencing side effects). Patients smoking >10 cigarettes/day: Start with 21 mg/day for six weeks, then 14 mg/day for two weeks, then 7 mg/day for two weeks. Patients smoking ≤10 cigarettes/day: Start with 14 mg/day for six weeks, then 7 mg/day for two weeks.
- Patients should be advised to completely stop smoking upon initiation of therapy.

MONITORING: No specific monitoring of note.

COST: $

SIDE EFFECTS:
Most common: Application site reactions (itching, burning, or redness), diarrhea, dyspepsia, abdominal pain.

MECHANISM, PHARMACOKINETICS, AND DRUG INTERACTIONS:
- Nicotinic-cholinergic receptor agonist.
- Metabolized primarily through liver as well as kidneys and lungs; t ½: 3–6 hours.
- Minimal risk for drug interactions. Successful cessation of smoking may increase serum levels of medications metabolized by CYP1A2 (eg, clozapine, olanzapine, theophylline), which is induced by hydrocarbons in smoke; nicotine itself has no effect.

EVIDENCE AND CLINICAL PEARLS:
- Nicotine patch therapy has been shown to be safe and effective for smoking cessation in adolescent smokers.
- One study in adolescents showed somewhat higher compliance with patch than with gum, but this may vary with patient preference.
- Start most patients who want to quit smoking on nicotine replacement therapy. Prescribe patch based on nicotine load: 1 ppd = 21 mg patch. Place it at the same time each day, usually in the morning. Start above the heart and rotate left around the body to prevent skin irritation. Use 0.5% cortisone cream for irritation/rash. Initial dose for four to eight weeks, then taper monthly or every two months. Advise no smoking—patients may note nausea or racing heart if they do.
- Patch may be worn for 16 or 24 hours. If craving upon awakening, wear patch for 24 hours; if vivid dreams or sleep disruptions occur, wear patch for 16 hours, then remove at bedtime.
- Do not cut patch; this causes rapid evaporation, making the patch useless.
- Up to 50% of patients will experience a local skin reaction, which is usually mild and self-limiting but may worsen with continued treatment. Local treatment with hydrocortisone cream 1% or triamcinolone cream 0.5% and rotating patch sites may help. In fewer than 5% of patients, such reactions require discontinuation.

FUN FACTS:
- In the US, nicotine patches and gum are available by prescription only for patients under 18 years (they are available over the counter for adults).
- In a particularly ironic scene in the dark comedy *Thank You for Smoking*, nicotine patches are used by antismoking "terrorists" to try to harm a marketing executive for Big Tobacco. The attempt fails because the executive already has a very high tolerance to nicotine, resulting in the headline "Smoking Saved My Life."

VARENICLINE (Chantix) Fact Sheet [G]

BOTTOM LINE:
Varenicline is the most effective tobacco cessation medication in adults but lacks data in adolescents, safety concerns aside. Psychiatric side effects are usually limited to insomnia or abnormal dreams. Dramatic reactions are possible but rare.

PEDIATRIC FDA INDICATIONS:
None.

ADULT FDA INDICATIONS:
Smoking cessation.

OFF-LABEL USES:
None.

DOSAGE FORMS:
Tablets (G): 0.5 mg, 1 mg.

DOSAGE GUIDANCE (ADULTS):
Start 0.5 mg QD x3 days, ↑ to 0.5 mg BID x4 days then ↑ to 1 mg BID for 11 weeks. Titrate slowly and take with food and a full glass of water to decrease GI upset. Start one week before target quit date; may consider setting a quit date up to 35 days after starting varenicline (to improve likelihood of abstinence).

MONITORING: No specific monitoring of note.

COST: $$$$

SIDE EFFECTS:
- Most common: Nausea, insomnia, headache, abnormal dreams, constipation, flatulence.
- Serious but rare: Neuropsychiatric events (eg, depression, suicidal thoughts, suicide, psychosis, hostility) reported, even without preexisting psychiatric disease. Warning recently revised as risk is lower than previously thought.

MECHANISM, PHARMACOKINETICS, AND DRUG INTERACTIONS:
- Nicotine receptor partial agonist.
- Excreted mostly unchanged with minimal hepatic (non-CYP450) metabolism; t ½: 24 hours.
- Potential lowered tolerance to alcohol, with psychiatric reactions. H2 blockers, quinolones, and trimethoprim may increase varenicline levels. Smoking cessation may alter pharmacokinetics of clozapine, olanzapine, theophylline, warfarin, insulin, and others.

EVIDENCE AND CLINICAL PEARLS:
- A 12-week randomized double-blind study in 157 smokers ages 14–21 found varenicline was well tolerated but did not differ from placebo in terms of abstinence. In those who did abstain, participants taking varenicline achieved abstinence earlier.
- Dual mechanism: partial agonist, mimicking nicotine effects on the brain and reducing withdrawal; also blocks nicotine binding, decreasing the reinforcing effect of smoking.
- If patient successfully quits smoking after 12 weeks, continue for another 12 weeks. If not successful in first 12 weeks, then discontinue and reassess factors contributing to failure.
- Similar quit rates as bupropion at six months (25%), but higher quit rates compared to bupropion at one year if a second 12-week course of varenicline is used.
- Can be combined with bupropion; use with nicotine replacement therapy likely to lead to increased side effects, particularly nausea, headache, vomiting, and dizziness.
- Recently touted for use in autism. Several case reports of improvement, but no other research exists.
- Discuss insomnia and vivid dreams with patients. Psychiatric side effects (eg, depression, suicidal ideation, and aggression) are likely caused by nicotine withdrawal, not Chantix.

FUN FACT:
The show *Saturday Night Live* aired a parody of a Chantix commercial suggesting that the side effects of *quitting* smoking could be dangerous (it's on YouTube).

Appendices

APPENDIX A: RATING SCALES

Standardized rating scales can be important tools during the clinical assessment and treatment process, helping to support or clarify diagnostic considerations, bring to light new areas of concern, and track symptoms. Rating scales are not diagnostic or intended to replace a thorough diagnostic interview. Always review the information provided about the scales you use to understand their benefits and limitations. We've included a list of commonly used scales that are in the public domain. See also www.thecarlatreport.com/the-carlat-child-psychiatry-report/using-clinical-scales-in-child-psychiatry/

If you are specifically looking for a diagnostic tool, consider the Kiddie Schedule for Affective Disorders and Schizophrenia (K-SADS), a semi-structured interview for ages 6–18 years that has been validated in research and clinical settings: www.pediatricbipolar.pitt.edu/sites/default/files/KSADS_DSM_5_SCREEN_Final.pdf

APPENDIX TABLE A: Rating Scales

Resource	Website
Abnormal Involuntary Movement Scale (AIMS) and Other Movement Scales (see Appendix B)	
Abnormal Involuntary Movement Scale (AIMS)	www.tinyurl.com/4m9hwm89
Yale Global Tic Severity Scale (YGTSS)	www.tinyurl.com/2pf3rwsw
The Massachusetts General Hospital Hair Pulling Scale	www.tinyurl.com/z78p6ujy
Trichotillomania Scale for Children, Child Version (TSC-C)	www.tinyurl.com/uyvhkvey
ADHD	
Child Attention Profile	www.tinyurl.com/bkjw4vpp
Conners' Parent Rating Scale—Revised	www.tinyurl.com/3253rara
SNAP-IV	www.tinyurl.com/523kuzu3
NICHQ Vanderbilt Assessment Scales	www.tinyurl.com/4mzumfds
Anxiety and Related Disorders	
Generalized Anxiety Disorder 7 (GAD-7)	www.tinyurl.com/yc5fy2f9
Children's Yale-Brown Obsessive Compulsive Scale (CY-BOCS)	www.tinyurl.com/43zsue6b
Screen for Child Anxiety Related Disorders (SCARED)	www.tinyurl.com/vyerrsy7
Spence Children's Anxiety Scale (SCAS)—Preschool Version	www.tinyurl.com/34at67ms
Autism and Related Challenges	
Childhood Autism Rating Scale (CARS)	www.tinyurl.com/5c78ywsj
Childhood Autism Spectrum Test (CAST)	www.tinyurl.com/bddjnva2
Greenspan Social-Emotional Growth Chart (part of the Bayley Scales, 0–42 months)	www.tinyurl.com/yuzkn6ty
Modified Checklist for Autism in Toddlers (M-CHAT)	www.tinyurl.com/yk3jr5ed
Parent's Observations of Social Interactions (POSI)	www.tinyurl.com/ycycyzbj
Eating Disorders	
Eating Attitudes Test (EAT-26)	www.tinyurl.com/yckxsux2
Eating Disorders in Youth—Questionnaire (EDY-Q; 8–13 years)	www.tinyurl.com/navfcjhb
Eating Disorder Screening Tool for Primary Care (ESP)	www.tinyurl.com/2s3cz3b6
Sick, Control, One, Fat, Food (SCOFF)	www.tinyurl.com/nnuvjv6z
The Pica, ARFID & Rumination Disorder Interview (PARDI)	www.tinyurl.com/mr2wx9r2
Mood Disorders	
The Brief Child Mania Rating Scale, Parent Version (B-CMRS-P)	www.tinyurl.com/yaxknfcp
Center for Epidemiological Studies Depression Scale for Children (CES-DC)	www.tinyurl.com/4eh6hfue
Childhood Depression Inventory (CDI) (the newer version, CDI-2, is a paid resource)	www.tinyurl.com/bddjjh54

Table A continued on the next page.

Resource	Website
Columbia-Suicide Severity Rating Scale (C-SSRS)	www.tinyurl.com/4p9rcycy
Mood Disorder Questionnaire (MDQ)	www.tinyurl.com/2p9bwzr2
Patient Health Questionnaire (PHQ-9)	www.tinyurl.com/4vka95vd
PTSD/Trauma	
Clinician-Administered PTSD Scale for DSM-5—Child/Adolescent Version (CAPS-CA-5)	www.tinyurl.com/2ubkpppx
Child and Adolescent Trauma Screen	www.tinyurl.com/54hy4etx
Life Events Checklist	www.tinyurl.com/3bucwh4x
Traumatic Events Screening Inventory for Children—Brief Form (TESI-C-Brief)	www.tinyurl.com/2p86t4tz
Traumatic Events Screening Inventory—Parent Report Revised (TESI-PRR)	www.tinyurl.com/39s7cumk
UCLA Brief COVID-19 Screen for Child/Adolescent PTSD	www.tinyurl.com/ykejp7s4
Young Child PTSD Checklist (YCPC)	www.tinyurl.com/52ydn5zu
Sleep	
Pediatric Sleep and Autism Clinical Global Impressions Scale	www.tinyurl.com/4uvpkf42
Pediatric Sleep Questionnaire	www.tinyurl.com/235sb6ku
Sleep Disturbance Scale for Children (SDSC)	www.tinyurl.com/3mkwxjtu
Substance Use	
Screening to Brief Intervention (S2BI)	www.tinyurl.com/3u7wrje8
CRAFFT	www.tinyurl.com/msrxsd3k
Clinical Opiate Withdrawal Scale (COWS)	www.tinyurl.com/yc4yfrhx
Clinical Institute Withdrawal Assessment of Alcohol Scale, Revised (CIWA-Ar)	www.tinyurl.com/ts3vnkfc
General and Miscellaneous	
Constipation: Bristol Stool Chart	www.tinyurl.com/4rwx7zyx
Patient-Reported Outcomes Measurement Information System (PROMIS measures)	www.tinyurl.com/yuy3yr9f
Pediatric Symptom Checklist-17 (PSC-17)	www.tinyurl.com/8km26brm

APPENDIX B: ABNORMAL INVOLUNTARY MOVEMENT SCALE (AIMS)

Overview

The Abnormal Involuntary Movement Scale (AIMS) is a rating scale designed in the 1970s to measure involuntary movements known as tardive dyskinesia (TD).

TD is a syndrome characterized by abnormal involuntary movements of the patient's face, mouth, trunk, or limbs. It affects 20%–30% of patients who have been treated for months or years with antipsychotic medications. Patients who are older, are heavy smokers, or have diabetes mellitus are at higher risk of developing TD. The movements of the patient's limbs and trunk are sometimes called choreoathetoid, which means a dance-like movement that repeats itself and has no rhythm. The AIMS test is used not only to detect TD but also to follow the severity of a patient's TD over time. The AIMS test is given every three to six months to monitor the patient for the development of TD.

The AIMS test can be completed in about 10 minutes. The test has a total of 12 items rating involuntary movements of various areas of the patient's body. Each item is rated on a five-point scale of severity: 0 (none), 1 (minimal), 2 (mild), 3 (moderate), or 4 (severe). Two of the 12 items are rated as yes or no and refer to dental status.

Many children and patients with developmental challenges may have difficulty collaborating with the clinician to do an AIMS screening. In those cases, we recommend that the clinician attempt the portions that are possible for the patient and record observations of the child and history from the family to assess the presence of abnormal involuntary movements.

Scoring

The total score on the AIMS test is not reported to the patient. A rating of 2 or higher on any section of the AIMS scale, however, is evidence of TD. If the patient has mild movements (score of 2) in two areas or moderate movements (score of 3) in one area, then he or she should be given a diagnosis of TD. The AIMS test is considered extremely reliable when it is given by experienced raters.

If the patient's test score suggests the diagnosis of TD, the clinician must consider whether the patient still needs to be on an antipsychotic medication. This question should be discussed with the patient and family. If the patient requires ongoing treatment with antipsychotic drugs, the dose can often be lowered. A lower dosage should result in a lower level of TD symptoms. Another option is to place the patient on a trial of clozapine (Clozaril).

APPENDIX TABLE B: Abnormal Involuntary Movement Scale (AIMS)

Instructions There are two parallel procedures, the examination procedure, which tells the patient what to do, and the scoring procedure, which tells the clinician how to rate what he or she observes.

Examination Procedure

Either before or after completing the examination procedure, observe the patient unobtrusively at rest (e.g., in the waiting room).

The chair to be used in this examination should be a hard, firm one without arms.

1. Ask the patient whether there is anything in his or her mouth (such as gum or candy) and, if so, to remove it.

2. Ask about the 'current' condition of the patient's teeth. Ask if he or she wears dentures. Ask whether teeth or dentures bother the patient 'now'.

3. Ask whether the patient notices any movements in his or her mouth, face, hands, or feet. If yes, ask the patient to describe them and to indicate to what extent they 'currently' bother the patient or interfere with activities.

4. Have the patient sit in the chair with hands on knees, legs slightly apart, and feet flat on floor. (Look at the entire body for movements while the patient is in this position.)

5. Ask the patient to sit with hands hanging unsupported – if male, between his legs, if female and wearing a dress, hanging over her knees. (Observe hands and other body areas).

6. Ask the patient to open his or her mouth. (Observe the tongue at rest within the mouth.) Do this twice.

7. Ask the patient to protrude his or her tongue. (Observe abnormalities of tongue movement.) Do this twice.

8. Ask the patient to tap his or her thumb with each finger as rapidly as possible for 10 to 15 seconds, first with right hand, then with left hand. (Observe facial and leg movements.) [±activated]

9. Flex and extend the patient's left and right arms, one at a time.

10. Ask the patient to stand up. (Observe the patient in profile. Observe all body areas again, hips included.)

11. Ask the patient to extend both arms out in front, palms down. (Observe trunk, legs, and mouth.) [activated]

12. Have the patient walk a few paces, turn, and walk back to the chair. (Observe hands and gait.) Do this twice. [activated]

Scoring Procedure

Complete the examination procedure before making ratings.

For the movement ratings (the first three categories below), rate the highest severity observed. 0 = none, 1 = minimal (may be extreme normal), 2 = mild, 3 = moderate, and 4 = severe. According to the original AIMS instructions, one point is subtracted if movements are seen **only on activation**, but not all investigators follow that convention.

Facial and Oral Movements

1. Muscles of facial expression, e.g., movements of forehead, eyebrows, periorbital area, cheeks. Include frowning, blinking, grimacing of upper face. 0 1 2 3 4

2. Lips and perioral area, e.g., puckering, pouting, smacking. 0 1 2 3 4

3. Jaw, e.g., biting, clenching, chewing, mouth opening, lateral movement. 0 1 2 3 4

4. Tongue. Rate only increase in movement both in and out of mouth, not inability to sustain movement. 0 1 2 3 4

Extremity Movements

5. Upper (arms, wrists, hands, fingers). Include movements that are choreic (rapid, objectively purposeless, irregular, spontaneous) or athetoid (slow, irregular, complex, serpentine). Do not include tremor (repetitive, regular, rhythmic movements). 0 1 2 3 4

6. Lower (legs, knees, ankles, toes), e.g., lateral knee movement, foot tapping, heel dropping, foot squirming, inversion and eversion of foot. 0 1 2 3 4

Trunk Movements

7. Neck, shoulders, hips, e.g., rocking, twisting, squirming, pelvic gyrations. Include diaphragmatic movements. 0 1 2 3 4

Global Judgments

8. Severity of abnormal movements. 0 1 2 3 4 based on the highest single score on the above items.

9. Incapacitation due to abnormal movements. 0 = none, normal 1 = minimal 2 = mild 3 = moderate 4 = severe

10. Patient's awareness of abnormal movements. 0 = no awareness 1 = aware, no distress 2 = aware, mild distress 3 = aware, moderate distress 4 = aware, severe distress

Dental Status

11. Current problems with teeth and/or dentures. 0 = no 1 = yes

12. Does patient usually wear dentures? 0 = no 1 = yes

Reproduced from Guy W. *ECDEU Assessment Manual for Psychopharmacology: Revised* (DHEW publication number ADM 76-338). Rockville, MD: US Department of Health, Education and Welfare, Public Health Service, Alcohol, Drug Abuse and Mental Health Administration, NIMH Psychopharmacology Research Branch, Division of Extramural Research Programs, 1976: 534–537.

Abnormal Involuntary Movement Scale (AIMS)

Public Health Service
Alcohol, Drug Abuse, and Mental Health Administration
National Institute of Mental Health

NAME: _____

DATE: _____

Prescribing Practitioner: _____

CODE   0=None
        1=Minimal, may be extreme normal
        2=Mild
        3=Moderate
        4-Severe

INSTRUCTIONS:
Complete Examination procedure (attachment d.)
Before making ratings

MOVEMENT RATINGS: Rate highest severity observed. Rate movements that occur upon activation one less than those observed spontaneously. Circle movement as well as code number that applies.		RATER	RATER	RATER	RATER
		Date	Date	Date	Date
Facial and Oral Movements	1. Muscles of Facial Expression eg, movements of forehead, eyebrows, periorbital area, cheeks, including frowning, blinking, smiling, grimacing	0 1 2 3 4	0 1 2 3 4	0 1 2 3 4	0 1 2 3 4
	2. Lips and Perioral Area eg, puckering, pouting, smacking	0 1 2 3 4	0 1 2 3 4	0 1 2 3 4	0 1 2 3 4
	3. Jaw eg, biting, clenching, chewing, mouth opening, lateral movement	0 1 2 3 4	0 1 2 3 4	0 1 2 3 4	0 1 2 3 4
	4. Tongue Rate only increases in movement both in and out of mouth, NOT inability to sustain movement. Darting in and out of mouth.	0 1 2 3 4	0 1 2 3 4	0 1 2 3 4	0 1 2 3 4
Extremity Movements	5. Upper (arms, wrists, hands, fingers) Include choreic movements (ie, rapid, objectively purposeless, irregular, spontaneous) athetoid movements (ie, slow, irregular, complex, serpentine). DO NOT INCLUDE TREMOR (ie, repetitive, regular, rhythmic)	0 1 2 3 4	0 1 2 3 4	0 1 2 3 4	0 1 2 3 4
	6. Lower (legs, knees, ankles, toes) eg, lateral knee movement, foot tapping, heel dropping, foot squirming, inversion and eversion of foot.	0 1 2 3 4	0 1 2 3 4	0 1 2 3 4	0 1 2 3 4
Trunk Movements	7. Neck, shoulders, hips eg, rocking, twisting, squirming, pelvic gyrations	0 1 2 3 4	0 1 2 3 4	0 1 2 3 4	0 1 2 3 4
Global Judgments	8. Severity of abnormal movements overall	0 1 2 3 4	0 1 2 3 4	0 1 2 3 4	0 1 2 3 4
	9. Incapacitation due to abnormal movements	0 1 2 3 4	0 1 2 3 4	0 1 2 3 4	0 1 2 3 4
	10. Patient's awareness of abnormal movements Rate only patient's report No awareness 0 Aware, no distress 1 Aware, mild distress 2 Aware, moderate distress 3 Aware, severe distress 4	0 1 2 3 4	0 1 2 3 4	0 1 2 3 4	0 1 2 3 4
Dental Status	11. Current problems with teeth and/or dentures?	No Yes	No Yes	No Yes	No Yes
	12. Are dentures usually worn?	No Yes	No Yes	No Yes	No Yes
	13. Edentia?	No Yes	No Yes	No Yes	No Yes
	14. Do movements disappear in sleep?	No Yes	No Yes	No Yes	No Yes

Appendices

Blood Pressure Levels for Boys by Age and Height Percentile

Age (Year)	BP Percentile ↓	Systolic BP (mmHg) ← Percentile of Height →							Diastolic BP (mmHg) ← Percentile of Height →						
		5th	10th	25th	50th	75th	90th	95th	5th	10th	25th	50th	75th	90th	95th
1	50th	80	81	83	85	87	88	89	34	35	36	37	38	39	39
	90th	94	95	97	99	100	102	103	49	50	51	52	53	53	54
	95th	98	99	101	103	104	106	106	54	54	55	56	57	58	58
	99th	105	106	108	110	112	113	114	61	62	63	64	65	66	66
2	50th	84	85	87	88	90	92	92	39	40	41	42	43	44	44
	90th	97	99	100	102	104	105	106	54	55	56	57	58	58	59
	95th	101	102	104	106	108	109	110	59	59	60	61	62	63	63
	99th	109	110	111	113	115	117	117	66	67	68	69	70	71	71
3	50th	86	87	89	91	93	94	95	44	44	45	46	47	48	48
	90th	100	101	103	105	107	108	109	59	59	60	61	62	63	63
	95th	104	105	107	109	110	112	113	63	63	64	65	66	67	67
	99th	111	112	114	116	118	119	120	71	71	72	73	74	75	75
4	50th	88	89	91	93	95	96	97	47	48	49	50	51	51	52
	90th	102	103	105	107	109	110	111	62	63	64	65	66	66	67
	95th	106	107	109	111	112	114	115	66	67	68	69	70	71	71
	99th	113	114	116	118	120	121	122	74	75	76	77	78	78	79
5	50th	90	91	93	95	96	98	98	50	51	52	53	54	55	55
	90th	104	105	106	108	110	111	112	65	66	67	68	69	69	70
	95th	108	109	110	112	114	115	116	69	70	71	72	73	74	74
	99th	115	116	118	120	121	123	123	77	78	79	80	81	81	82
6	50th	91	92	94	96	98	99	100	53	53	54	55	56	57	57
	90th	105	106	108	110	111	113	113	68	68	69	70	71	72	72
	95th	109	110	112	114	115	117	117	72	72	73	74	75	76	76
	99th	116	117	119	121	123	124	125	80	80	81	82	83	84	84
7	50th	92	94	95	97	99	100	101	55	55	56	57	58	59	59
	90th	106	107	109	111	113	114	115	70	70	71	72	73	74	74
	95th	110	111	113	115	117	118	119	74	74	75	76	77	78	78
	99th	117	118	120	122	124	125	126	82	82	83	84	85	86	86
8	50th	94	95	97	99	100	102	102	56	57	58	59	60	60	61
	90th	107	109	110	112	114	115	116	71	72	72	73	74	75	76
	95th	111	112	114	116	118	119	120	75	76	77	78	79	79	80
	99th	119	120	122	123	125	127	127	83	84	85	86	87	87	88
9	50th	95	96	98	100	102	103	104	57	58	59	60	61	61	62
	90th	109	110	112	114	115	117	118	72	73	74	75	76	76	77
	95th	113	114	116	118	119	121	121	76	77	78	79	80	81	81
	99th	120	121	123	125	127	128	129	84	85	86	87	88	88	89
10	50th	97	98	100	102	103	105	106	58	59	60	61	61	62	63
	90th	111	112	114	115	117	119	119	73	73	74	75	76	77	78
	95th	115	116	117	119	121	122	123	77	78	79	80	81	81	82
	99th	122	123	125	127	128	130	130	85	86	86	88	88	89	90

Source: www.nhlbi.nih.gov

Blood Pressure Levels for Boys by Age and Height Percentile (Continued)

Age (Year)	BP Percentile ↓	Systolic BP (mmHg) ← Percentile of Height →							Diastolic BP (mmHg) ← Percentile of Height →						
		5th	10th	25th	50th	75th	90th	95th	5th	10th	25th	50th	75th	90th	95th
11	50th	99	100	102	104	105	107	107	59	59	60	61	62	63	63
	90th	113	114	115	117	119	120	121	74	74	75	76	77	78	78
	95th	117	118	119	121	123	124	125	78	78	79	80	81	82	82
	99th	124	125	127	129	130	132	132	86	86	87	88	89	90	90
12	50th	101	102	104	106	108	109	110	59	60	61	62	63	63	64
	90th	115	116	118	120	121	123	123	74	75	75	76	77	78	79
	95th	119	120	122	123	125	127	127	78	79	80	81	82	82	83
	99th	126	127	129	131	133	134	135	86	87	88	89	90	90	91
13	50th	104	105	106	108	110	111	112	60	60	61	62	63	64	64
	90th	117	118	120	122	124	125	126	75	75	76	77	78	79	79
	95th	121	122	124	126	128	129	130	79	79	80	81	82	83	83
	99th	128	130	131	133	135	136	137	87	87	88	89	90	91	91
14	50th	106	107	109	111	113	114	115	60	61	62	63	64	65	65
	90th	120	121	123	125	126	128	128	75	76	77	78	79	79	80
	95th	124	125	127	128	130	132	132	80	80	81	82	83	84	84
	99th	131	132	134	136	138	139	140	87	88	89	90	91	92	92
15	50th	109	110	112	113	115	117	117	61	62	63	64	65	66	66
	90th	122	124	125	127	129	130	131	76	77	78	79	80	80	81
	95th	126	127	129	131	133	134	135	81	81	82	83	84	85	85
	99th	134	135	136	138	140	142	142	88	89	90	91	92	93	93
16	50th	111	112	114	116	118	119	120	63	63	64	65	66	67	67
	90th	125	126	128	130	131	133	134	78	78	79	80	81	82	82
	95th	129	130	132	134	135	137	137	82	83	83	84	85	86	87
	99th	136	137	139	141	143	144	145	90	90	91	92	93	94	94
17	50th	114	115	116	118	120	121	122	65	66	66	67	68	69	70
	90th	127	128	130	132	134	135	136	80	80	81	82	83	84	84
	95th	131	132	134	136	138	139	140	84	85	86	87	87	88	89
	99th	139	140	141	143	145	146	147	92	93	93	94	95	96	97

BP, blood pressure

* The 90th percentile is 1.28 SD, 95th percentile is 1.645 SD, and the 99th percentile is 2.326 SD over the mean.

For research purposes, the standard deviations in Appendix Table B–1 allow one to compute BP Z-scores and percentiles for boys with height percentiles given in Table 3 (i.e., the 5th,10th, 25th, 50th, 75th, 90th, and 95th percentiles). These height percentiles must be converted to height Z-scores given by (5% = -1.645; 10% = -1.28; 25% = -0.68; 50% = 0; 75% = 0.68; 90% = 1.28%; 95% = 1.645) and then computed according to the methodology in steps 2–4 described in Appendix B. For children with height percentiles other than these, follow steps 1–4 as described in Appendix B.

Source: www.nhlbi.nih.gov

Appendices

Blood Pressure Levels for Girls by Age and Height Percentile

Age (Year)	BP Percentile ↓	Systolic BP (mmHg) ← Percentile of Height →							Diastolic BP (mmHg) ← Percentile of Height →						
		5th	10th	25th	50th	75th	90th	95th	5th	10th	25th	50th	75th	90th	95th
1	50th	83	84	85	86	88	89	90	38	39	39	40	41	41	42
	90th	97	97	98	100	101	102	103	52	53	53	54	55	55	56
	95th	100	101	102	104	105	106	107	56	57	57	58	59	59	60
	99th	108	108	109	111	112	113	114	64	64	65	65	66	67	67
2	50th	85	85	87	88	89	91	91	43	44	44	45	46	46	47
	90th	98	99	100	101	103	104	105	57	58	58	59	60	61	61
	95th	102	103	104	105	107	108	109	61	62	62	63	64	65	65
	99th	109	110	111	112	114	115	116	69	69	70	70	71	72	72
3	50th	86	87	88	89	91	92	93	47	48	48	49	50	50	51
	90th	100	100	102	103	104	106	106	61	62	62	63	64	64	65
	95th	104	104	105	107	108	109	110	65	66	66	67	68	68	69
	99th	111	111	113	114	115	116	117	73	73	74	74	75	76	76
4	50th	88	88	90	91	92	94	94	50	50	51	52	52	53	54
	90th	101	102	103	104	106	107	108	64	64	65	66	67	67	68
	95th	105	106	107	108	110	111	112	68	68	69	70	71	71	72
	99th	112	113	114	115	117	118	119	76	76	76	77	78	79	79
5	50th	89	90	91	93	94	95	96	52	53	53	54	55	55	56
	90th	103	103	105	106	107	109	109	66	67	67	68	69	69	70
	95th	107	107	108	110	111	112	113	70	71	71	72	73	73	74
	99th	114	114	116	117	118	120	120	78	78	79	79	80	81	81
6	50th	91	92	93	94	96	97	98	54	54	55	56	56	57	58
	90th	104	105	106	108	109	110	111	68	68	69	70	70	71	72
	95th	108	109	110	111	113	114	115	72	72	73	74	74	75	76
	99th	115	116	117	119	120	121	122	80	80	80	81	82	83	83
7	50th	93	93	95	96	97	99	99	55	56	56	57	58	58	59
	90th	106	107	108	109	111	112	113	69	70	70	71	72	72	73
	95th	110	111	112	113	115	116	116	73	74	74	75	76	76	77
	99th	117	118	119	120	122	123	124	81	81	82	82	83	84	84
8	50th	95	95	96	98	99	100	101	57	57	57	58	59	60	60
	90th	108	109	110	111	113	114	114	71	71	71	72	73	74	74
	95th	112	112	114	115	116	118	118	75	75	75	76	77	78	78
	99th	119	120	121	122	123	125	125	82	82	83	83	84	85	86
9	50th	96	97	98	100	101	102	103	58	58	58	59	60	61	61
	90th	110	110	112	113	114	116	116	72	72	72	73	74	75	75
	95th	114	114	115	117	118	119	120	76	76	76	77	78	79	79
	99th	121	121	123	124	125	127	127	83	83	84	84	85	86	87
10	50th	98	99	100	102	103	104	105	59	59	59	60	61	62	62
	90th	112	112	114	115	116	118	118	73	73	73	74	75	76	76
	95th	116	116	117	119	120	121	122	77	77	77	78	79	80	80
	99th	123	123	125	126	127	129	129	84	84	85	86	86	87	88

Source: www.nhlbi.nih.gov

Blood Pressure Levels for Girls by Age and Height Percentile (Continued)

Age (Year)	BP Percentile ↓	Systolic BP (mmHg) ← Percentile of Height →							Diastolic BP (mmHg) ← Percentile of Height →						
		5th	10th	25th	50th	75th	90th	95th	5th	10th	25th	50th	75th	90th	95th
11	50th	100	101	102	103	105	106	107	60	60	60	61	62	63	63
	90th	114	114	116	117	118	119	120	74	74	74	75	76	77	77
	95th	118	118	119	121	122	123	124	78	78	78	79	80	81	81
	99th	125	125	126	128	129	130	131	85	85	86	87	87	88	89
12	50th	102	103	104	105	107	108	109	61	61	61	62	63	64	64
	90th	116	116	117	119	120	121	122	75	75	75	76	77	78	78
	95th	119	120	121	123	124	125	126	79	79	79	80	81	82	82
	99th	127	127	128	130	131	132	133	86	86	87	88	88	89	90
13	50th	104	105	106	107	109	110	110	62	62	62	63	64	65	65
	90th	117	118	119	121	122	123	124	76	76	76	77	78	79	79
	95th	121	122	123	124	126	127	128	80	80	80	81	82	83	83
	99th	128	129	130	132	133	134	135	87	87	88	89	89	90	91
14	50th	106	106	107	109	110	111	112	63	63	63	64	65	66	66
	90th	119	120	121	122	124	125	125	77	77	77	78	79	80	80
	95th	123	123	125	126	127	129	129	81	81	81	82	83	84	84
	99th	130	131	132	133	135	136	136	88	88	89	90	90	91	92
15	50th	107	108	109	110	111	113	113	64	64	64	65	66	67	67
	90th	120	121	122	123	125	126	127	78	78	78	79	80	81	81
	95th	124	125	126	127	129	130	131	82	82	82	83	84	85	85
	99th	131	132	133	134	136	137	138	89	89	90	91	91	92	93
16	50th	108	108	110	111	112	114	114	64	64	65	66	66	67	68
	90th	121	122	123	124	126	127	128	78	78	79	80	81	81	82
	95th	125	126	127	128	130	131	132	82	82	83	84	85	85	86
	99th	132	133	134	135	137	138	139	90	90	90	91	92	93	93
17	50th	108	109	110	111	113	114	115	64	65	65	66	67	67	68
	90th	122	122	123	125	126	127	128	78	79	79	80	81	81	82
	95th	125	126	127	129	130	131	132	82	83	83	84	85	85	86
	99th	133	133	134	136	137	138	139	90	90	91	91	92	93	93

BP, blood pressure

* The 90th percentile is 1.28 SD, 95th percentile is 1.645 SD, and the 99th percentile is 2.326 SD over the mean.

For research purposes, the standard deviations in Appendix Table B–1 allow one to compute BP Z-scores and percentiles for girls with height percentiles given in Table 4 (i.e., the 5th, 10th, 25th, 50th, 75th, 90th, and 95th percentiles). These height percentiles must be converted to height Z-scores given by (5% = -1.645; 10% = -1.28; 25% = -0.68; 50% = 0; 75% = 0.68; 90% = 1.28%; 95% = 1.645) and then computed according to the methodology in steps 2–4 described in Appendix B. For children with height percentiles other than these, follow steps 1–4 as described in Appendix B.

Source: www.nhlbi.nih.gov

Appendices

APPENDIX D: GROWTH, BODY MASS INDEX, AND HEAD CIRCUMFERENCE CHARTS

Limitations and Cautions on Using Body Mass Index (BMI)

Remember that while BMI is a useful measure for population-based studies, it does not reflect the health of an individual the way blood pressure or hemoglobin A1c do. Weight stigma and fat shaming permeate the health care field, and people experience discrimination based on their BMI values. We recommend using BMI only in the narrowest clinical sense, such as to gauge the use of a GLP-1 agonist if you must use a weight-producing antipsychotic. For more information on this topic, see *The Carlat Child Psychiatry Report,* July/August/September 2022.

Appendix D continued on the next page.

2 to 20 years: Boys
Body mass index-for-age percentiles

NAME _____

RECORD # _____

Date	Age	Weight	Stature	BMI*	Comments

*To Calculate BMI: Weight (kg) ÷ Stature (cm) ÷ Stature (cm) x 10,000
or Weight (lb) ÷ Stature (in) ÷ Stature (in) x 703

BMI

AGE (YEARS)

kg/m²

Published May 30, 2000 (modified 10/16/00).
SOURCE: Developed by the National Center for Health Statistics in collaboration with
the National Center for Chronic Disease Prevention and Health Promotion (2000).

SAFER · HEALTHIER · PEOPLE™

Source: www.cdc.gov/growthcharts

2 to 20 years: Girls
Body mass index-for-age percentiles

NAME _____

RECORD # _____

Date	Age	Weight	Stature	BMI*	Comments

*To Calculate BMI: Weight (kg) ÷ Stature (cm) ÷ Stature (cm) x 10,000
or Weight (lb) ÷ Stature (in) ÷ Stature (in) x 703

AGE (YEARS)

Published May 30, 2000 (modified 10/16/00).
SOURCE: Developed by the National Center for Health Statistics in collaboration with
the National Center for Chronic Disease Prevention and Health Promotion (2000).

Source: www.cdc.gov/growthcharts

SAFER · HEALTHIER · PEOPLE™

Published May 30, 2000 (modified 11/21/00).
SOURCE: Developed by the National Center for Health Statistics in collaboration with
the National Center for Chronic Disease Prevention and Health Promotion (2000).

Source: www.cdc.gov/growthcharts

2 to 20 years: Girls
Stature-for-age and Weight-for-age percentiles

NAME _____

RECORD # _____

Published May 30, 2000 (modified 11/21/00).
SOURCE: Developed by the National Center for Health Statistics in collaboration with
the National Center for Chronic Disease Prevention and Health Promotion (2000).

SAFER · HEALTHIER · PEOPLE™

Source: www.cdc.gov/growthcharts

Head Circumference

While we do not encourage substantial psychotropic prescribing in infants and young children, we've included the CDC head circumference charts here because they come in handy during initial and some follow-up evaluations, particularly for young children with suspected developmental challenges who may have microcephaly or macrocephaly.

CDC Growth Charts: United States

Head circumference-for-age percentiles: Boys, birth to 36 months

Age (months)

Published May 30, 2000.
SOURCE: Developed by the National Center for Health Statistics in collaboration with
the National Center for Chronic Disease Prevention and Health Promotion (2000).

CDC
SAFER · HEALTHIER · PEOPLE™

CDC Growth Charts: United States

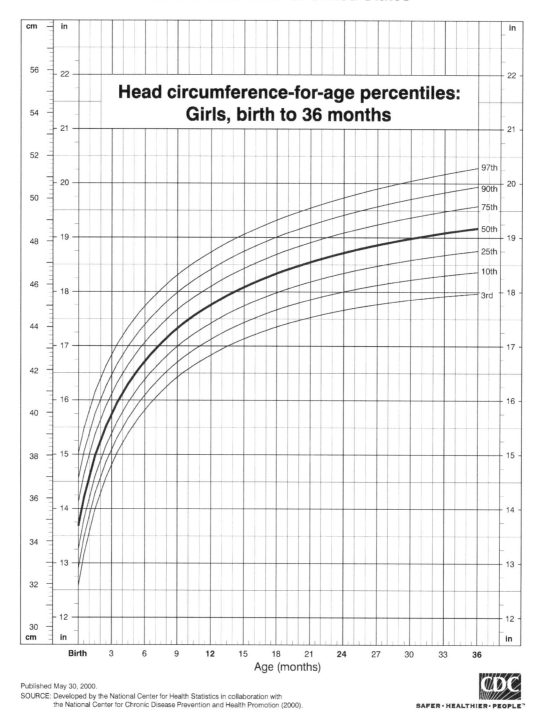

Head circumference-for-age percentiles: Girls, birth to 36 months

Published May 30, 2000.
SOURCE: Developed by the National Center for Health Statistics in collaboration with
the National Center for Chronic Disease Prevention and Health Promotion (2000).

SAFER · HEALTHIER · PEOPLE™

APPENDIX E: LAB MONITORING FOR PSYCHIATRIC MEDICATIONS

This is a short and sweet table listing the medications that most psychiatrists would agree require lab monitoring. Our recommendations are quite abbreviated, and we haven't spelled out whether you should order labs before or after starting the medications, nor how you should do follow-up monitoring. There's just too much variation in practice for us to give authoritative detailed guidelines. These medications are mainly here to jog your memory, so you don't forget to at least consider what type of monitoring to do.

APPENDIX TABLE E: Lab Monitoring for Psychiatric Medications

Medications	Recommended Laboratory Tests
Acamprosate	BUN/creatinine if renal impairment is suspected
Amantadine	BUN/creatinine if renal impairment is suspected
Antipsychotics (see also clozapine, paliperidone below)	BMI, fasting glucose and/or HbA1c, fasting lipids; prolactin if symptoms and routine for risperidone, paliperidone, haloperidol, thiothixene, and fluphenazine; ECG especially chlorpromazine, thioridazine, ziprasidone; consider periodic slit-lamp examinations to screen for cataracts; periodic AIMS for TD screening[1]
Atomoxetine	LFTs
Carbamazepine	Complete blood count (CBC), sodium, LFTs, pregnancy test, HLA-B*1502 in those of Asian descent[2], carbamazepine level (at least 3 days on stable dose, trough level, 12 hours after last dose); target: 4–12 mcg/mL
Citalopram	ECG if cardiac disease, dose ≥40 mg/day
Clomipramine	Clomipramine/norclomipramine levels (at least 5 days on stable dose, trough level, 12 hours after last dose); target: 220–500 ng/mL
Clozapine	BMI, fasting glucose and/or HbA1c, fasting lipids, CBC (REMS system required in US for neutrophil monitoring); clozapine/norclozapine serum level (at least 3 days on stable dose, trough level, 12 hours after last dose); target: >350 ng/mL; toxicity: >700 ng/mL
Desvenlafaxine	Periodic BP
Deutetrabenazine	ECG if cardiac disease
Disulfiram	LFTs if liver disease is suspected
Duloxetine	LFTs if liver disease is suspected[3]
Gabapentin	BUN/creatinine if renal impairment is suspected
Levomilnacipran	Periodic BP/pulse rate
Lithium	BMI, TSH, BUN/creatinine[4], pregnancy test, ECG if cardiac disease; lithium serum level (at least 5 days on stable dose, trough level, 12 hours after last dose); target: 0.8–1.2 mEq/L (acute mania) and 0.6–1.0 mEq/L (maintenance)
Methadone	ECG if cardiac disease
Mirtazapine	BMI, fasting glucose and lipids
Naltrexone	LFTs if liver disease is suspected
Oxcarbazepine	Sodium, HLA-B*1502 in those of Asian descent[2]
Paliperidone	BUN/creatinine; BMI, fasting glucose and/or HbA1c, fasting lipids; prolactin if symptoms and routine for risperidone, paliperidone, haloperidol, thiothixene, and fluphenazine; ECG; consider periodic slit-lamp examinations to screen for cataracts; periodic AIMS for TD screening
Pregabalin	BUN/creatinine if renal impairment is suspected
SSRIs	Sodium in elderly if fatigue, dizziness, confusion
Stimulants	Periodic BP/P, height and weight, ECG if cardiac disease
Topiramate	Bicarbonate
Tricyclic antidepressants	ECG if cardiac disease
Valbenazine	ECG if cardiac disease
Valproic acid	BMI, LFTs, CBC for platelets, pregnancy test, ammonia if confusion, amylase and lipase if symptomatic for possible pancreatitis; valproic acid serum level (at least 3 days on stable dose, trough level, 12 hours after last dose with IR or 21–24 hours with ER); target: 50–125 mcg/mL
Venlafaxine	Periodic BP

[1] Some guidelines recommend monitoring glucose and lipids with all SGAs.

[2] HLA-B*1502 is a gene that increases the risk of developing toxic epidermal necrolysis (TEN) and Stevens-Johnson syndrome (SJS) in response to taking carbamazepine. Asians, especially the Han Chinese, are much more likely to have the gene than other populations.

[3] Duloxetine should not be prescribed in patients with significant alcohol use or evidence of chronic liver disease as it can lead to hepatic failure in rare cases (Cymbalta prescribing information). While the manufacturer does not recommend baseline LFTs for all patients, some clinicians do so anyway to be extra cautious.

[4] The serum creatinine is used to compute the estimated glomerular filtration rate (eGFR), a more precise measure of kidney functioning. Increasingly, laboratory test results include the estimated GFR. You can calculate it yourself using an online calculator: www.niddk.nih.gov/health-information/communication-programs/nkdep/laboratory-evaluation/glomerular-filtration-rate-calculators

APPENDIX F: GUIDELINES FOR INFORMED CONSENT

We recommend that you include the following elements in your informed consent process:

- Diagnoses or working diagnoses.

- Target symptoms, prioritized.

- Proposed medication plan, including name of medication, dosage, timing, and plans for adjusting.

- Specific rationale (benefits) and risks (side effects), including any black box warnings.

- Alternatives to medication, including no medication.

- FDA-approved use vs off-label use of medication. Families need to know that while doctors are allowed to use medications however they see fit, many medications are not approved by the FDA for children and are officially considered experimental. The discussion should include some information on common off-label uses, a sense of the supporting research and rationale, and a plan to manage problems if they arise.

- Any additional regulations, if applicable (eg, state or institutional requirements regarding use or follow-up).

- Cost of care, including medications, brand names vs generics, follow-up visits, and cost-saving strategies.

- Monitoring plan, including labs and frequency of follow-up visits.

- Concurrent treatment and intervention: therapies, school plans, etc.

In addition, consider the following while speaking with patients and families:

- Check your state laws for age of consent for mental health care, and specifically for medication treatment.

- For children whose parents are divorced, check the custody papers for information on shared health care decision making. For example, can one parent consent to medication if the other parent objects? There may also be a difference in decision making authority during routine vs emergency situations.

- Consider assent: What will you tell the child, and to what extent can the child be a partner in the process?

- Agree to stay in contact as needed, and specify how to reach you or your coverage.

- Finally, remember that informed consent is an ongoing process that supports good care. Periodically review the treatment plan, documenting your review and noting any changes to the plan if applicable.

APPENDIX G: MENTAL HEALTH APPS

There has been an exponential growth in apps over the last several years, many touting benefits for various mental and medical health reasons. A few have been FDA approved with research to support their use, while the majority have not. Some are free, while others require a subscription or have add-on charges. It is important to consider the privacy policies (or lack thereof) of these apps—as they are not subject to HIPAA law, many lack basic security measures for users, and the majority profit from the collection of personal data. The apps listed in our table are available through the Apple (iOS) app store unless otherwise noted. A comprehensive website of mental health apps can be found here: https://mindapps.org/Home

APPENDIX TABLE G: Mental Health Apps

Calming and Meditation
Breathe2Relax
Desk Yogi
iMindfulness (Android devices only)
Mindfulness Daily[1]
Stop, Breathe & Think (Android devices only)
UCLA Mindful
Calm
Headspace
Insight Timer
Smiling Mind
Ten Percent Happier
CBT
CBT Tools for Healthy Living (Android devices only)
MindShift CBT
Disaster and Trauma
PFA Mobile
Psychological First Aid (PFA) Tutorial
SAMHSA Disaster Response
Mood Disorders and Suicidality
DBSA Wellness Tracker[2]
Mood Tracker[4]
IntelliCare[3]
Virtual Hope Box
Sleep
CBT-i Coach
SnoreLab
Substance Use
Sober Time
Miscellaneous
Medisafe[5]
Migraine Buddy
Peers®

[1] Mindfulness Daily is a free online course available at www.soundstrue.com/products/mindfulness-daily

[2] DBSA Wellness Tracker is a suite of free tools available at www.dbsalliance.org/wellness/wellness-toolbox/wellness-tracker/

[3] IntelliCare is a series of NIH-funded, CBT-based apps for anxiety, depression, and insomnia—individual modules are available in most app stores, and the full suite is available at https://intellicare.cbits.northwestern.edu

[4] Mood Tracker is a free browser-based app (with paid options) available at www.moodtracker.com

[5] Medisafe provides medication reminders

APPENDIX H: DRUG INTERACTIONS IN PSYCHIATRY

Drug interactions can be one of the most challenging aspects of psychopharmacology. Here we've provided a brief review. For more information, see *Prescribing Psychotropics: From Drug Interactions to Pharmacogenetics* (Carlat Publishing, 2021).

Today's psychiatrists often use complex medication regimens, while patients frequently take medications for multiple comorbidities. It's impossible to keep track of every facet of a patient's regimen, but it is important (1) to understand basic concepts of drug-drug interactions, (2) to know where to find information regarding such interactions, and (3) to know which interactions may be clinically relevant. This review is pertinent to both general and child psychiatry; however, see the General Tips chapter for specific thoughts on age-related differences in children's drug metabolism.

The majority of interactions in psychiatry will not result in a serious outcome. Many interactions may result in decreased efficacy or increased adverse effects, which we can easily avoid through our existing knowledge of how the drugs work. However, we often do not have data on side effects and interactions in children.

First, let's review some basic concepts. A drug interaction occurs when the pharmacologic action of one drug is altered by the co-administration of another drug. The two major types of drug interactions are **pharmacodynamic** (what the drug does to the body) and **pharmacokinetic** (what the body does to the drug). Pharmacodynamic interactions impact the effects of the drug at the target site. Pharmacokinetic interactions, on the other hand, impact the amount of time the drug stays in the body and its distribution to active sites.

Pharmacodynamic interactions take place at the level of neurotransmitters and receptors. For example, quetiapine (Seroquel) makes people sleepy, probably by blocking histamine receptors. Clonazepam (Klonopin) also makes people sleepy, by stimulating GABA receptors. Combine the two, and patients become *really* sleepy. Pharmacodynamic interactions may also cause two drugs to *oppose* one another. Many of the dementia medications, for example, increase acetylcholine levels, while many psychiatric medications have primary (eg, benztropine) or secondary (eg, clozapine) anticholinergic effects. Giving both together may negate the beneficial effects of the dementia medication.

Some notable—and potentially dangerous—pharmacodynamic interactions in psychiatry include serotonin syndrome (too many serotonergic agents used together); the MAOI-type hypertensive crisis (MAOIs taken with foods high in tyramine); and arrhythmia-causing combinations (cumulative increases in QT interval that may cause life-threatening arrhythmias, such as torsades de pointes). We often try to avoid these problems by doing things like lowering doses or choosing alternative medications. In such cases, we're trying to avoid pharmacodynamic interactions.

Pharmacokinetic interactions are harder to predict, since they are often unintuitive and unrelated to the pharmacologic action of drugs. Pharmacokinetic interactions depend on where and when two or more drugs come in contact during drug processing. Drugs can interact with one another at four junctures:

- Absorption (getting the drug into the bloodstream)

- Distribution (ferrying drugs to different tissues once they've been absorbed)

- Excretion (sending drugs into the sewage system)

- Metabolism (dismantling drugs into simpler components)

We'll discuss each one in turn, focusing on some common examples in psychopharmacology.

Absorption. Drug-food, rather than drug-drug, interactions are most relevant during absorption. For example, ziprasidone (Geodon) and lurasidone (Latuda) absorption are both decreased by 50%–60% when taken without food, which is why we should instruct our patients to take these drugs after a full meal. Food also speeds absorption of sertraline (Zoloft) and quetiapine, but only by 25% or so, usually not enough to be clinically relevant. Meanwhile, food famously *slows* absorption of erectile dysfunction drugs such as sildenafil (Viagra) and vardenafil (Levitra)—but not tadalafil (Cialis).

Distribution. Valproic acid (Depakote) is highly protein-bound, and only the unbound portion (the "free fraction") of the drug has a therapeutic effect. Aspirin is also highly protein-bound, so if your patient combines the two drugs, the aspirin will kick some of the valproic acid off its protein—mainly albumin—which would cause the free fraction of the drug to increase. Standard valproic acid levels in the lab usually do not distinguish between free and bound fractions, so a serum level might be normal even while the actual functioning valproic acid level is very high—and this could cause side effects. One way to check for this interaction is to order a free valproate level; the normal therapeutic range is about 5–10 mcg/mL, much less than the total valproic acid therapeutic range of about 40–100 mcg/mL.

Excretion. Lithium, unlike almost all other drugs in psychiatry, is not metabolized. Instead, it is excreted unchanged in the urine. Because of this, liver disease does not affect lithium levels, but changes in kidney function do. Caffeine, for example, speeds up kidney function and can reduce lithium levels. On the other hand, ibuprofen (along with other NSAIDs) and ACE inhibitors decrease lithium excretion, increase lithium levels, and could cause toxic effects. Other psychiatric medications that are excreted by the kidneys and not metabolized by the liver are gabapentin (Neurontin), pregabalin (Lyrica), and paliperidone (Invega).

Metabolism. Most drug-drug interactions take place in the liver, where drugs are processed in order to render them water-soluble so that the body can excrete them via the urine or feces. There are two phases of liver metabolism. Phase I involves the famous cytochrome P-450 enzymes, or CYP450. These enzymes attack drugs in a variety of ways, such as hydroxylation (adding a hydroxyl group), dealkylation (taking away an alkyl group), and several others. Unfortunately for those of us trying to remember drug interactions, there are many subfamilies of CYP450 enzymes: CYP1A2, 2B6, 2C9, 2C19, 2D6, 3A4, and several others. Phase II metabolism continues the process of biotransformation, relying mainly on glucuronidation—which is rarely a factor in drug interactions relevant to psychiatric practice.

Practical Implications of Drug-Drug Interactions

To understand drug-drug interactions, you'll need to refamiliarize yourself with some basic terms. Drugs are **substrates** of specific enzymes (meaning a medication relies on one or more specific enzymatic pathways for metabolism). An **inhibitor** is a drug that binds more tightly to an enzyme than the usual substrate and prevents the enzyme from doing its job; as a result, the substrate for that enzyme gets stuck in a game of musical chairs as it scurries around looking for a free enzyme system to break it down. Since this drug is not getting metabolized as quickly as it otherwise would (the inhibitor is preventing it from doing so), its serum levels become higher than expected. On the other hand, **inducers** stimulate the production of extra enzymes. With more enzymes around, the substrate for that enzyme is broken down more rapidly, leading to lower serum drug levels.

Now that you know the basics, how can you most efficiently apply them to your practice? Here are some suggestions:

- Identify the 10 drugs that you most commonly prescribe, and memorize the major drug interactions for each one.

- Be particularly vigilant if your patient is taking antidepressants, antipsychotics, antibiotics, antiretrovirals, or older anticonvulsants—all of which have a high likelihood of significant drug interactions.

- Recognize the drugs that have a narrow therapeutic window (ie, a toxic dose that is not much higher than the therapeutic dose). Commonly used drugs with narrow therapeutic windows include lithium, carbamazepine (Tegretol), warfarin (Coumadin), digoxin (Lanoxin), phenytoin (Dilantin), and phenobarbital.

- Recognize drugs that cause serious side effects and outcomes if their serum levels are significantly increased or decreased (eg, oral contraceptives, lamotrigine, clozapine, TCAs, warfarin).

- Remember that drugs with long half-lives, such as aripiprazole (Abilify) or diazepam (Valium), can be particularly troublesome when involved in drug interactions, because metabolic inhibitors—or hepatic dysfunction—can make them ultra-long-lasting. Be cautious with any new or rarely prescribed drugs: Neither you nor anybody else has had much experience with them, and unreported drug interactions can appear.

- Remember that the risk of drug interactions can increase exponentially as the number of drugs increases. Setting a threshold to check for interactions is helpful (eg, any patient on three or more drugs).

Another important concern with drug interactions is timing. *Inhibition* happens quickly. It can occur with the first dose of a medication and can subside rapidly, depending on the inhibitor's half-life. Generally, the inhibition will stop after five half-lives of the inhibitor drug. Inhibition is also dose-related; the higher the dose of the inhibitor, the more likely or significant the drug interaction. On the other hand, for *induction* to occur, the body has to synthesize more CYP450 enzymes, which can take up to four weeks. This accounts for the delayed "auto-induction" of carbamazepine. Likewise, for induction to subside, these extra enzymes need to be broken down, a process that can also take several weeks. As a general rule, any drug prescribed with its inhibitor should be started at half the usual dose and titrated more slowly. Conversely, a drug prescribed with its inducer may need to be dosed higher after the few weeks it takes for induction to occur.

Useful References for Drug Interactions

It's ideal to have a useful resource to look up interaction information. Keeping track of interactions has become less daunting with the advent of free software from companies like Epocrates (www.epocrates.com) and Medscape (www.medscape.com), which allow you to check for potential interactions among all possible combinations of drugs.

But there are various problems with the computerized databases you'll find at these sites or in your electronic prescribing system (if you have one). For one, the databases tend to be overly inclusive, often listing every conceivable interaction, no matter how unlikely. As an example, citalopram (Celexa), an SSRI considered by most of us to be a pretty safe choice in combination with just about any drug, looks pretty dangerous in the Epocrates database. Moreover, these databases are often populated with drug-class information rather than medication-specific information, making important nuances unavailable to the user. That's where your clinical judgment and experience come in!

Free

- Medscape (www.medscape.com/druginfo/druginterchecker)
- Epocrates (www.epocrates.com; you'll need to register first)
- Drugs.com (www.drugs.com/drug_interactions.html)

- Indiana University CYP450 interaction table (www.medicine.iupui.edu/clinpharm/ddis)
- RxList (www.rxlist.com)

Not free

- Lexicomp (www.wolterskluwer.com/en/solutions/lexicomp), $119 for one-year subscription

We also provide a table on the following pages for your reference (adapted from *The Carlat Psychiatry Report,* February 2011).

Appendix H continued on the next page.

APPENDIX TABLE H: Drug Interactions in Psychiatry

CYP450 Family	Inducers	Inhibitors	Substrates ("Victim" Drugs)	Symptoms When Induced	Symptoms When Inhibited
1A2	Armodafinil Carbamazepine Cigarette smoke Modafinil Omeprazole Rifampin Ritonavir St. John's wort	Ciprofloxacin Fluvoxamine Melatonin Norfloxacin	Asenapine	Loss of efficacy (psychosis)	Insomnia/EPS
			Caffeine	Withdrawal headaches	Jitteriness
			Clozapine	Loss of efficacy (psychosis)	Seizures/sedation/anticholinergic effects
			Duloxetine	Loss of efficacy (depression)	Increased blood pressure
			Fluvoxamine	Loss of efficacy (depression/OCD)	GI/sedation
			Melatonin	Loss of efficacy (insomnia)	Sedation
			Mirtazapine	Loss of efficacy (depression)	Sedation
			Olanzapine	Loss of efficacy (psychosis)	Sedation
			Ramelteon	Loss of efficacy (insomnia)	Sedation
			Tasimelteon	Loss of efficacy (insomnia)	Sedation
			Thiothixene	Loss of efficacy (psychosis)	EPS
			Trifluoperazine	Loss of efficacy (psychosis)	EPS
2B6	Carbamazepine Phenobarbital Phenytoin Rifampin	Clopidogrel Ketoconazole Ticlopidine	Bupropion	Loss of efficacy (depression)	Seizures/jitteriness/insomnia
			Methadone	Opioid withdrawal	CNS and respiratory depression
			Selegiline	Loss of efficacy (depression)	Insomnia/diarrhea
2C9	Barbiturates Carbamazepine Rifampin St. John's wort	Fluconazole Fluoxetine Fluvoxamine Isoniazid Metronidazole	Methadone	Opioid withdrawal	CNS and respiratory depression
			NSAIDs	Loss of pain control	GI effects
			Oral hypoglycemics	Loss of glycemic control	Hypoglycemia
			Warfarin	Loss of anticoagulant efficacy	Increased bleeding
2C19	Barbiturates Carbamazepine Phenytoin Rifampin	Armodafinil Fluconazole Fluoxetine Fluvoxamine Modafinil Oxcarbazepine	Barbiturates	Loss of efficacy (insomnia/anxiety/seizures)	Sedation/barbiturate intoxication
			Citalopram	Loss of efficacy (depression/anxiety)	GI effects
			Diazepam	Loss of efficacy (insomnia/anxiety/seizures)	Sedation/BZD intoxication
			Doxepin	Loss of efficacy (depression/anxiety/insomnia)	Seizures/arrhythmia/anticholinergic effects
			Escitalopram	Loss of efficacy (depression/anxiety)	GI effects
			Methadone	Opioid withdrawal	CNS and respiratory depression
			Sertraline	Loss of efficacy (depression/anxiety)	GI effects

( ) indicates less potent inhibitory effect, therefore generally less of a risk except at higher dose

CYP450 Family	Inducers	Inhibitors	Substrates ("Victim" Drugs)	Symptoms When Induced	Symptoms When Inhibited
2D6	Not inducible	Asenapine Bupropion Duloxetine Fluoxetine Haloperidol Methadone Paroxetine Thioridazine Venlafaxine	Amphetamine	N/A	Insomnia/decreased appetite
			Aripiprazole	N/A	Akathisia/sedation
			Atomoxetine	N/A	GI/constipation
			Brexpiprazole	N/A	Akathisia/sedation
			Chlorpromazine	N/A	Seizures/sedation/anticholinergic effects
			Clozapine	N/A	Seizures/sedation/anticholinergic effects
			Codeine/hydrocodone	N/A	Less/no analgesia (not converted to morphine)
			Deutetrabenazine	N/A	Sedation/QT prolongation
			Dextroamphetamine	N/A	Insomnia/decreased appetite
			Diphenhydramine	N/A	Sedation/anticholinergic effects
			Donepezil	N/A	GI effects
			Doxepin	N/A	Sedation/anticholinergic effects
			Doxylamine	N/A	Sedation/anticholinergic effects
			Duloxetine	N/A	Increased BP
			Fluoxetine	N/A	GI effects
			Fluphenazine	N/A	EPS
			Fluvoxamine	N/A	GI effects/sedation
			Galantamine	N/A	GI effects
			Haloperidol	N/A	EPS
			Iloperidone	N/A	Tachycardia/hypotension/stiffness
			Lisdexamfetamine (prodrug of dextroamphetamine)	N/A	Insomnia/decreased appetite
			Loxapine	N/A	EPS/sedation
			Methamphetamine	N/A	Insomnia/decreased appetite
			Mirtazapine	N/A	Somnolence
			Mixed amphetamine salts	N/A	Insomnia/decreased appetite
			Paroxetine	N/A	GI effects/anticholinergic effects/sedation
			Perphenazine	N/A	EPS/sedation
			Pitolisant	N/A	Insomnia/anxiety
			Propranolol	N/A	Decreased BP/pulse
			Risperidone	N/A	EPS/orthostasis

( ) indicates less potent inhibitory effect, therefore generally less of a risk except at higher dose

Appendices

CYP450 Family	Inducers	Inhibitors	Substrates ("Victim" Drugs)	Symptoms When Induced	Symptoms When Inhibited
2D6	Not inducible	Asenapine Bupropion Duloxetine Fluoxetine Haloperidol Methadone Paroxetine Thioridazine Venlafaxine	Thioridazine	N/A	Seizures/sedation/anticholinergic effects/QT prolongation
			Trazodone	N/A	Sedation
			Tricyclics	N/A	Seizures/arrhythmia/anticholinergic effects
			Valbenazine	N/A	Sedation/QT prolongation
			Venlafaxine	N/A	GI effects
			Vortioxetine	N/A	GI effects
3A4	Armodafinil Barbiturates Carbamazepine Modafinil Oxcarbazepine Phenytoin Rifampin St. John's wort	Clarithromycin Fluconazole Fluvoxamine Grapefruit juice Ketoconazole Nefazodone Protease inhibitors (including Paxlovid)	Alprazolam	Loss of efficacy (insomnia/anxiety/seizures)	Sedation/BZD intoxication
			Aripiprazole	Loss of efficacy (psychosis)	Akathisia/sedation
			Armodafinil	Loss of efficacy (narcolepsy)	Insomnia/increased pulse
			Avanafil	Loss of efficacy (sexual dysfunction)	Headache/flushing/prolonged erection
			Brexpiprazole	Loss of efficacy (psychosis)	Akathisia/sedation
			Buprenorphine	Opioid withdrawal	CNS and respiratory depression
			Buspirone	Loss of efficacy (anxiety)	GI effects/jitteriness
			Calcium channel blockers	Loss of efficacy (hypertension)	Hypotension
			Carbamazepine	Loss of efficacy/seizures	Sedation/arrhythmia
			Cariprazine	Loss of efficacy (psychosis)	Akathisia/sedation
			Citalopram	Loss of efficacy (depression/anxiety)	GI effects
			Clonazepam	Loss of efficacy (insomnia/anxiety/seizures)	Sedation/BZD intoxication
			Clozapine	Loss of efficacy (psychosis)	Seizures/sedation/anticholinergic effects
			Diazepam	Loss of efficacy (insomnia/anxiety/seizures)	Sedation/BZD intoxication
			Donepezil	Loss of efficacy (dementia)	GI effects
			Escitalopram	Loss of efficacy (depression/anxiety)	GI effects
			Eszopiclone	Loss of efficacy (insomnia)	Sedation/confusion
			Flibanserin	Loss of efficacy (sexual desire)	Nausea/dizziness/sedation
			Flurazepam	Loss of efficacy (insomnia)	Sedation/BZD intoxication
			Galantamine	Loss of efficacy (dementia)	GI effects
			Guanfacine	Loss of efficacy (ADHD)	Sedation/dry mouth/dizziness
			Iloperidone	Loss of efficacy (psychosis)	Sedation/dizziness
			Lemborexant	Loss of efficacy (insomnia)	Sedation/confusion
			Levomilnacipran	Loss of efficacy (depression)	GI effects

( ) indicates less potent inhibitory effect, therefore generally less of a risk except at higher dose

CYP450 Family	Inducers	Inhibitors	Substrates ("Victim" Drugs)	Symptoms When Induced	Symptoms When Inhibited
3A4	Armodafinil Barbiturates Carbamazepine Modafinil Oxcarbazepine Phenytoin Rifampin St. John's wort (Topiramate)	Clarithromycin Fluconazole Fluvoxamine Grapefruit juice Ketoconazole Protease inhibitors (including Paxlovid)	Loxapine	Loss of efficacy (psychosis)	EPS/sedation
			Lurasidone	Loss of efficacy (psychosis)	Sedation/akathisia
			Methadone	Opioid withdrawal	CNS and respiratory depression
			Mirtazapine	Loss of efficacy (depression/insomnia)	Somnolence
			Modafinil	Loss of efficacy (narcolepsy)	Insomnia/increased pulse
			Nefazodone	Loss of efficacy (depression)	Sedation/orthostasis
			Oral contraceptives	Loss of efficacy (pregnancy)	GI effects
			Pimavanserin	Loss of efficacy (psychosis)	Nausea/confusion
			Pitolisant	Loss of efficacy (excessive daytime sedation)	Insomnia/anxiety
			Quetiapine	Loss of efficacy (psychosis)	Sedation/orthostasis
			Sildenafil	Loss of efficacy (sexual dysfunction)	Headache/flushing/prolonged erection
			Statins (not pravastatin)	Loss of efficacy (hyperlipidemia)	Rhabdomyolysis
			Suvorexant	Loss of efficacy (insomnia)	Sedation/confusion
			Tadalafil	Loss of efficacy (sexual dysfunction)	Headache/flushing/prolonged erection
			Tasimelteon	Loss of efficacy (insomnia)	Sedation
			Tiagabine	Loss of efficacy (seizures)	Dizziness/somnolence/difficulty concentrating
			Trazodone	Loss of efficacy (insomnia)	Sedation/orthostasis
			Triazolam	Loss of efficacy (insomnia/anxiety/seizures)	Sedation/BZD intoxication
			Tricyclics	Loss of efficacy (depression/anxiety)	Seizures/arrhythmia/anticholinergic effects
			Vardenafil	Loss of efficacy (sexual dysfunction)	Headache/flushing/prolonged erection
			Vilazodone	Loss of efficacy (depression/anxiety)	GI effects
			Zaleplon	Loss of efficacy (insomnia)	Sedation/confusion
			Ziprasidone	Loss of efficacy (psychosis)	Sedation/akathisia
			Zolpidem	Loss of efficacy (insomnia)	Sedation/confusion

( ) indicates less potent inhibitory effect, therefore generally less of a risk except at higher dose

APPENDIX I: MEDICATIONS IN PREGNANCY AND LACTATION RISK INFORMATION

(By way of explanation, we elected to include this appendix because some of our teen patients become pregnant, as do some of the parents of our pediatric patients, during their mental health treatment. Many of us treat patients of childbearing age in any case.)

Determining the risk of medications in pregnancy used to be a simple matter of looking up a drug's pregnancy categorization in the *PDR*. This ranged from category "A," which is the lowest risk, to "X," which means the drug is contraindicated in pregnancy. But this ABCDX system provided very little practical or clinically useful information. In 2014, the FDA came up with a new system of labeling, which requires descriptive subsections on different aspects of pregnancy and lactation, and omits the letter categories—though you'll still see the old system in use for drugs approved before 2015.

Pregnancy presents a unique problem to the psychiatrist. Contrary to what many may think or assume, pregnancy does not protect a patient from an acute episode, a recurrence, or an exacerbation of psychiatric illness. Withholding medications during pregnancy can *sometimes* be an appropriate option, but is generally not recommended. Ever-mounting research demonstrates that the mental well-being of the patient during pregnancy and in the postpartum period (and beyond) is critical to the emotional development of the child. And since all psychotropic medications cross the placenta to at least *some* degree, their potential effects on the fetus, on labor and delivery, and on the neonate must be considered and balanced with the risk of *not* treating the pregnant patient with medication (see *The Carlat Psychiatry Report,* July/August 2016, for an overview). A similar risk-benefit assessment must be considered in the case of patients who wish to breastfeed their children, as psychotropic medications are excreted into breast milk to varying degrees.

One of us (TP) is a pharmacist specializing in psychopharmacology who is commonly consulted by psychiatrists to provide updated information on the safety of medications in pregnancy and breastfeeding. It is a difficult task, because the quantity and quality of data vary greatly. The accompanying table was developed by pulling together a variety of sources, including isolated case reports, case series, birth registries, retrospective surveys, prospective comparative cohort studies, case control studies, and meta-analyses. Making judgments about which medication to use—or not use—in a pregnant or lactating patient is a delicate balancing act, involving an assessment of the severity of the underlying illness versus the uncertainties inherent in prescribing medications with limited data.

When reading the table, keep the following in mind: In the general US population, the baseline rate of major malformations is between 1% and 4%, depending on the population studied and the definitions of "malformations" used. If treatment is necessary, monotherapy with the lowest *effective* dose and for the shortest duration is prudent. Safety data are generally more robust with older agents, and for that reason older agents—with a few key exceptions—are more preferable than newer drugs with less established safety profiles.

Almost all drugs enter breast milk. The exposure to the infant is described as a percentage of the parent's dose—that is, how much of the weight-adjusted dose is actually excreted into the breast milk. When less than 10% of a parent's dose of medication is excreted into the breast milk, the medication is generally considered compatible with breastfeeding (with some exceptions) since these low serum levels are unlikely to lead to adverse effects in the infant.

While the table summarizes the current knowledge about psychotropic medications in pregnancy and lactation, information in this area is constantly evolving. If you regularly treat patients of childbearing age, we suggest that you keep up with new data, consult with experts, and use resources such as:

- Organization of Teratology Information Specialists (www.mothertobaby.org; 866-626-6847)

- The National Library of Medicine's LactMed database, peer reviewed and updated monthly (www.ncbi.nlm.nih.gov/books/NBK501922)

- MGH Center for Women's Mental Health (www.womensmentalhealth.org)

- The CDC's wide range of offerings (www.cdc.gov/pregnancy/meds)

If you don't mind paying a fee (or if you are a trainee and have free access), you can also check out www.reprotox.org, an online database of summaries. Drug labeling, which has become more detailed as of 2015, can be another source of information. These resources, along with our table, provide information based upon the available evidence (or lack thereof). However, the ultimate clinical decision always comes down to careful and individualized consideration between the physician, patient, and family.

Additional References

- Besag FM. ADHD treatment and pregnancy. *Drug Saf* 2014;37(6):397–408.

- Betcher HK and Wisner KL. Psychotropic treatment during pregnancy: Research synthesis and clinical care principles. *J Womens Health (Larchmt)* 2020;29(3):310–318.

- Chisolm MS et al. Management of psychotropic drugs during pregnancy. *BMJ* 2016;352:h5918.

- Khan SJ et al. Bipolar disorder in pregnancy and postpartum: Principles of management. *Curr Psychiatry Rep* 2016;18(2):13.

Appendices

- McLafferty LP et al. Guidelines for the management of pregnant women with substance use disorders. *Psychosomatics* 2016;57(2):115–130.

- Muzik M et al. Use of antidepressants during pregnancy? What to consider when weighing treatment with antidepressants against untreated depression. *Matern Child Health J* 2016;20(11):2268–2279.

- Ornoy A et al. Antidepressants, antipsychotics, and mood stabilizers in pregnancy: What do we know and how should we treat pregnant women with depression? *Birth Defects Res* 2017:109(12):933–956.

- Oyebode F et al. Psychotropics in pregnancy: Safety and other considerations. *Pharmacol Ther* 2012;135(1):71–77.

- Payne JL. Psychiatric medication use in pregnancy and breastfeeding. *Obstet Gynecol Clin North Am* 2021;48(1):131–149.

- Payne JL. Psychopharmacology in pregnancy and breastfeeding. *Med Clin North Am* 2019;103(4):629–650.

- Raffi ER et al. Safety of psychotropic medications during pregnancy. *Clin Perinatol* 2019;46(2):215–234.

- Raidoo S and Kaneshiro B. Contraception counseling for adolescents. *Curr Opin Obstet Gynecol* 2017;29(5):310–315.

- Rowe H et al. Maternal medication, drug use, and breastfeeding. *Child Adolesc Psychiatr Clin N Am* 2015;24(1):1–20.

- Sachs HC et al. The transfer of drugs and therapeutics into human breast milk: An update on selected topics. *Pediatrics* 2013;132(3):e796–e809.

- Vigod S et al. Depression in pregnancy. *BMJ* 2016;352:i547.

Appendix I continued on the next page.

APPENDIX TABLE I: Medications in Pregnancy and Lactation Risk Information

Medication	Pregnancy	Breastfeeding	Recommendations
Anxiolytics/Hypnotics			
Benzodiazepines (various agents)	Possible increased incidence of cleft lip or palate (with first-trimester exposure); floppy infant syndrome (with exposure just before delivery); neonatal withdrawal syndrome; lower Apgar scores	Excretion varies with different benzodiazepines, but it is always less than 10%. Excessive sedation in infant, lethargy with consequent feeding difficulty and weight loss reported.	Try to avoid use in first trimester and late in pregnancy (although intermittent use less likely to induce withdrawal symptoms in neonate). Lorazepam (Ativan) may be best in class to use due to lack of active metabolites and relatively shorter half-life. Monitor sedation in breastfed infants; use of shorter-acting agents preferred.
Buspirone (BuSpar)	Fewer data; difficult to determine risks	Low to undetectable infant levels reported	Due to lack of data, other agents with larger safety database should be considered first; avoid in pregnancy. Likely safe in breastfeeding.
Diphenhydramine (Benadryl)	Fairly consistent data show lack of associated malformations	Larger doses or more prolonged use may cause adverse effects in the infant	Considered to be the safest hypnotic in pregnancy and breastfeeding
Non-benzodiazepines: eszopiclone (Lunesta), zaleplon (Sonata), zolpidem (Ambien)	Fewer data show no increased risk of malformations	Relatively low levels in breast milk. Most data are with zolpidem. Zolpidem is relatively hydrophilic and excreted rapidly; therefore, may be favored.	Reserve for second-line use due to paucity of data. If unavoidable, use zolpidem at lowest dose possible.
Suvorexant (Belsomra), lemborexant (Dayvigo)	No data	No data	Best to use other agents with data and longer record of experience
Trazodone	Fewer data show no increased risk of malformations	<1% excretion; not expected to cause adverse effects in breastfed infants	Probably safe in pregnancy and breastfeeding
Mood Stabilizers			
Carbamazepine (Tegretol)	Rate of major malformation reported to be 2.2%–7.9%. Neural tube defects (0.5%–1%), craniofacial defects, cardiovascular malformations, and hypospadias reported.	Relatively high levels in breast milk but with few adverse effects reported. Sedation, poor sucking, withdrawal reactions, and 3 cases of hepatic dysfunction have been reported.	Avoid if possible. High-dose (4 mg) folic acid supplementation recommended if use unavoidable.
Lamotrigine (Lamictal)	Rate of major malformations reported to be 1%–5.6%. Increased risk of oral clefts (0.4%).	Based on limited data, thought to be safe; however, infant exposure can be high and can vary widely (reports of 18%–60% of maternal concentrations); monitor infant. Relatively high infant exposure (22.7%); avoid or exercise caution.	Considered to be the safest of the anticonvulsants in pregnancy, though good safety data are sparse. Serum levels should be monitored; levels usually decrease over course of pregnancy.
Lithium (Eskalith, Lithobid)	Rate of major malformations reported to be 4%–12%. Increased risk of cardiovascular malformation, Ebstein's anomaly; risk is lower than previously thought (0.05%–0.1%). Increased maternal risk of diabetes, polyhydramnios, thyroid dysfunction during pregnancy.	30%–50% excretion; not recommended due to high risk of toxicity	Avoid, particularly in first trimester. Check serum levels and thyroid function frequently during pregnancy. Changes in metabolism and total body water necessitate frequent dose adjustment, particularly in third trimester. Avoid in breastfeeding if possible.
Oxcarbazepine (Trileptal)	Unlike carbamazepine, there is no epoxide metabolite formed, so oxcarbazepine may be less teratogenic; a Danish study showed no increased risk of major malformation. However, data with oxcarbazepine are limited.	Limited information suggests oxcarbazepine would not be expected to cause adverse effects in breastfed infants, especially if the infant is older than 2 months. Monitor infant for drowsiness, adequate weight gain, and developmental milestones, especially in younger, exclusively breastfed infants and when using combinations of anticonvulsants.	Use caution until more data available

Medication	Pregnancy	Breastfeeding	Recommendations
Valproate (Depakote)	Most teratogenic of all mood stabilizers, with a 6.2%–20.3% rate of congenital malformations, with neural tube defects most prominent. Teratogenic effects are dose-related with greatest risk at doses >1000 mg per day. Recently, exposure linked to autism.	Relatively low excretion (0.68%); considered compatible with breastfeeding	Best to avoid in pregnancy unless absolutely required. High-dose (4 mg) folic acid supplementation recommended if use unavoidable. Safe in breastfeeding.
Antipsychotics			
Second-generation	Fewer data available, most showing no increased risk of malformations. Maternal hyperglycemia, impaired glucose tolerance, and weight gain may lead to maternal complications. Large-for-gestational-age infants reported. Floppy infant syndrome reported in clozapine exposure; monitor neutrophils in neonate for 6 months.	Excretion low, usually <3%, with exception of clozapine (Clozaril), which is seen in relatively high concentrations in breast milk	Overall, relatively safe in pregnancy; not treating serious mental illness in pregnancy poses greater risk. Most data with risperidone, olanzapine, quetiapine. Avoid clozapine in breastfeeding if possible.
First-generation	No increased risk of malformations seen with high-potency agents. Small increase in risk with low-potency agents such as chlorpromazine (Thorazine). Transient extrapyramidal side effects; sedation; withdrawal symptoms in neonates.	Relatively low excretion reported although little data available. Sedation and Parkinsonism effects possible in breastfed infants.	Haloperidol (Haldol), fluphenazine (Prolixin) favored during pregnancy because of long history of safe use and fewer hypotensive, anticholinergic, and antihistaminergic effects. Limited data in breastfeeding; relatively safe.
Antidepressants			
Bupropion (Wellbutrin)	No increased risk of malformation shown thus far	<1% excretion with no adverse outcomes reported	Well-characterized and considered reasonable option. May also help with smoking cessation during pregnancy.
Duloxetine (Cymbalta)	Little data	No published data, though exposure is low	Other agents with more data favored
Levomilnacipran (Fetzima)	No data	No published data	Other agents with more data favored
Mirtazapine (Remeron)	Sparse data, but one small study suggests no increased rate of major malformation	Low excretion; compatible with breastfeeding	May be useful also for pregnancy-associated emesis, insomnia
SSRIs	Controversial data regarding cardiovascular malformation with first-trimester paroxetine (Paxil) exposure. Larger and more recent studies show no overall increased risk for malformations with SSRIs. Conflicting reports with some studies showing decreased gestational age, low birth weight, poor neonatal adaptation, low Apgar scores (some of which could be due to underlying depression or anxiety). Conflicting reports regarding SSRI use in later pregnancy and persistent pulmonary hypertension (PPHN). Neonatal toxicity reported as transient jitteriness, tremulousness, and tachypnea. No problems detected in behavioral or cognitive development—greatest data with fluoxetine (Prozac).	Relatively low excretion, varies by agent: Citalopram (Celexa): 5%–10% Fluoxetine: 3%–9% Fluvoxamine (Luvox): <2% Paroxetine: <4% Sertraline (Zoloft): <2%	Best-studied and most-used class of psychotropics in pregnancy. Relatively safe in pregnancy; avoid paroxetine if possible. Sertraline results in lowest fetal drug exposure and lowest (undetectable) levels in breastfed infants; may be considered favored SSRI. Paroxetine use most controversial. Fluoxetine less favored for breastfeeding due to long half-life and active metabolite; disturbed sleep, colic, irritability, poor feeding reported.
Tricyclics	Relatively large database; recent meta-analysis of 300,000 live births revealed no increased risk of malformations. Neonatal anticholinergic effects. Transient neonatal withdrawal symptoms reported.	<1%–5% excretion; appear relatively safe during breastfeeding, with possible exception of doxepin	Well characterized and considered reasonable options. Desipramine (Norpramin), nortriptyline (Pamelor) preferred due to lower anticholinergic and orthostatic hypotension risks. Monitor baby for sedation in breastfeeding.

Medication	Pregnancy	Breastfeeding	Recommendations
Venlafaxine/desvenlafaxine (Pristiq)	Earlier data regarding major malformations reassuring, but a more recent study suggested a possible association with birth defects; additional studies needed. Increased maternal blood pressure may be a concern during pregnancy, particularly at higher doses.	2%–9.2% excretion; no adverse outcomes reported	Other agents with more data favored
Vilazodone (Viibryd)	No data	No published data	Other agents with more data favored
Vortioxetine (Trintellix)	No data	No published data	Other agents with more data favored
Stimulants			
Amphetamines and methylphenidate	No apparent congenital malformations; may constrict blood flow to placenta, which reduces oxygen flow to developing fetus. May cause premature delivery, small-for-gestational-age and low-birth-weight babies; however, data inconclusive. Neonatal withdrawal possible.	0.2% excreted into breast milk; adverse effects usually not observed	Caution in pregnancy due to possibility of vasoconstriction and ability to disrupt blood flow to the fetus. Likely safe in breastfeeding.

APPENDIX J: SCHEDULES OF CONTROLLED SUBSTANCES

In 1970, under the Controlled Substance Act, the FDA created classification schedules that organize drugs into groups based on their risk of abuse or harm. There are five classifications of controlled substances (Schedule I, II, III, IV, and V), and drugs with the highest risk-to-benefit ratio are considered Schedule I drugs. Most drugs used in psychiatry (antidepressants, antipsychotics, etc) are not scheduled at all. Some of us get confused about whether the most restricted drugs are Schedule I or V. Here's a mnemonic: The number 1 looks like a needle, and a needle is used to inject heroin—which is the prototypical Schedule I drug. The DEA's more comprehensive and regularly updated listing can be found here: www.tinyurl.com/3xck57xs

Prescription drug monitoring programs (PDMPs) are searchable databases that can help prescribers identify potential abuse or diversion of controlled substances. If you prescribe controlled substances like benzodiazepines and stimulants, it's a good idea to learn about your state's PDMP laws, consider your search results in the context of all available information, and watch for regulatory changes over the next few years. For example, since October 2, 2018, prescribers in California must check the state CURES database before prescribing controlled substances. To find your state's program, check with the PDMP Training and Technical Assistance Center: www.pdmpassist.org/content/state-pdmp-websites

APPENDIX TABLE J: Schedules of Controlled Substances

Schedule	Description	Prescribing Implications	Some Examples
I	No accepted medical use, high potential for abuse, illegal to possess or use	Can't be prescribed at all (with the exception of medical marijuana in some states)	Heroin, LSD, ecstasy, and others Marijuana (though legalized in some states, it is still illegal at the federal level)
II	High potential for abuse, but legal for medical use	Can be prescribed only 1 month at a time, cannot be refilled, cannot be called in	All psychostimulants, such as amphetamine and methylphenidate Opiates that are especially potent, such as oxycodone, fentanyl, and others Vicodin (hydrocodone and acetaminophen)—recently reclassified from Schedule III to Schedule II
III	Lower potential for abuse than Schedule I or II, but still pretty abusable	Can be refilled up to 5 times (no more than 6 months), can be called in	Anabolic steroids Barbiturates Dronabinol (Marinol) Esketamine (Spravato) Ketamine Suboxone (buprenorphine/naloxone) Xyrem (sodium oxybate) Zywav (mixed-salts oxybate)
IV	Lower potential for abuse than Schedule III	Can be refilled up to 5 times (no more than 6 months), can be called in	All benzodiazepines (eg, clonazepam, lorazepam, etc) Various hypnotics, such as lemborexant (Dayvigo), zolpidem, zaleplon, and suvorexant (Belsomra) Wake-promoting agents, like modafinil, armodafinil, and solriamfetol (Sunosi) Carisoprodol (Soma) Lorcaserin (Belviq), an anti-obesity drug Tramadol (Ultram)
V	Lowest potential for abuse	Can be refilled as many times as prescriber chooses (eg, for 1 year or more), can be called in	Pregabalin (Lyrica) Cough preparations with small amounts of codeine, such as Robitussin AC Antidiarrheal Lomotil (diphenoxylate/atropine)

An updated and more complete list of the schedules is published annually in Title 21 *Code of Federal Regulations* and can be found here: www.deadiversion.usdoj.gov/schedules/orangebook/c_cs_alpha.pdf

APPENDIX K: PHARMACOGENETIC TESTING RECOMMENDATIONS

The Basics

Variations in patients' genetic profiles can affect how they respond to medications. While the actual clinical importance of this phenomenon is not yet clear, it's likely that variations in pharmacokinetic genes have some effect on serum levels of medications in many patients. Based on these CYP450 polymorphisms, individuals are categorized in different ways with respect to specific enzymes:

- **Extensive metabolizers:** Otherwise known as "normal" metabolizers, these people have normally active CYP450 genes on both chromosomes, meaning that they see an average level of drug in the body.

- **Intermediate metabolizers:** These people metabolize drugs a bit more slowly than extensive metabolizers, but not dramatically so.

- **Poor metabolizers:** These people carry inactive or partially active CYP450 genes, and therefore metabolize drugs significantly more slowly than extensive metabolizers. This may result in more side effects since serum drug levels are higher.

- **Ultrarapid metabolizers:** With extra copies of certain genes, these people metabolize drugs more quickly than extensive metabolizers, sometimes requiring unusually high doses of medications to achieve a therapeutic level.

There are also variations in pharmacodynamic genes that might increase or decrease the efficacy of drugs, but the evidence for this effect is less robust than for pharmacokinetic effects.

Pharmacogenetic Testing in Clinical Practice

The science of pharmacogenetic testing is complex, and the limited existing research calls into question the accuracy of both the tests and the clinical guidance from the commercial test kits flooding the market.

At this time, we lack robust evidence to recommend any pharmacogenetic tests such as Genesight, Genecept, or CNSDose (for more information, see *The Carlat Psychiatry Report,* March 2017, and *The Carlat Child Psychiatry Report,* January 2021). The FDA nevertheless has recommendations for pharmacogenetic testing relevant to specific psychotropic drugs, which we have included in Appendix Table K.

The FDA often recommends lowering the starting dose in patients who are poor metabolizers. For example, in aripiprazole's label, you'll read: "Dosing recommendation in patients who are classified as CYP450 2D6 poor metabolizers (PM): The aripiprazole dose in PM patients should initially be reduced to one-half (50%) of the usual dose and then adjusted to achieve a favorable clinical response."

While the FDA does not specifically ask you to order genetic testing, you will not know whether your patient is a poor metabolizer unless someone has ordered it. Therefore, you could make a case for selectively ordering CYP450 testing to ensure you dose drugs in accordance with FDA labeling. Whether you do this is a judgment call; most of us are content to skip the genetic testing, and instead choose to start most medications at a low dose and titrate up gradually in order to prevent side effects.

Appendix K continued on the next page.

APPENDIX TABLE K: FDA Label Information Relevant to Pharmacogenetic Testing for Psychiatric Drugs

Medication	FDA Recommendations	Clinical Rationale
Amphetamines Aripiprazole Atomoxetine Brexpiprazole Deutetrabenazine Iloperidone Perphenazine Pimozide Pitolisant Tetrabenazine Thioridazine Valbenazine Venlafaxine Vortioxetine	Reduce dose in CYP2D6 PMs[1]	Usual starting dose is too high in PMs, so start lower and increase gradually
Amitriptyline Clomipramine Clozapine Desipramine Doxepin Imipramine Nortriptyline Protriptyline Trimipramine	Monitor levels in CYP2D6 PMs	These medications, most of which are tricyclic antidepressants, can cause life-threatening side effects if levels are too high; consider monitoring serum levels in PMs
Carbamazepine Oxcarbazepine	Avoid or use cautiously in individuals with the HLA-B*1502 allele (applicable to those of Asian descent)	Risk of serious rashes such as Stevens-Johnson syndrome
Citalopram	Maximum recommended daily dose of 20 mg (rather than 40 mg) for CYP2C19 PMs	Risk of QT prolongation and cardiac arrhythmia
Pimozide	In CYP2D6 PMs, dose should not exceed 4 mg/day in adults	Risk of QT prolongation and cardiac arrhythmia
Thioridazine	Contraindicated in CYP2D6 PMs, due to risk of QT prolongation	Risk of QT prolongation and cardiac arrhythmia

[1]PM = poor metabolizer

Source: www.fda.gov/medical-devices/precision-medicine/table-pharmacogenetic-associations

Index

NOTE: Trade names are capitalized, bolded page numbers are for fact sheets, and non-bolded page numbers are for quick-scan tables and general prescribing information.

Printed in the USA
CPSIA information can be obtained
at www.ICGtesting.com
LVHW070813151023
761014LV00081B/1780